DATE DUE

GAYLORD			PRINTED IN U.S A.

AN ABSTRACT FOR ACTION

AN
ABSTRACT FOR ACTION

JEROME P. LYSAUGHT, Ed.D.

Director

*National Commission for the study of
Nursing and Nursing Education*

McGRAW-HILL BOOK COMPANY

A Blakiston Publication

*New York, St. Louis, San Francisco, Düsseldorf, London,
Mexico, Panama, Sydney, Toronto*

AN ABSTRACT FOR ACTION

Library of Congress Catalog Card Number 73-126176

   34567890   MAMM   7987654321

ISBN 07-045797-2 CL
      045798-0 SF

*This book was set in Optima by John C. Meyer & Son, and
printed on permanent paper and bound by The Maple
Press Company. The designer was Paula Tuerk. The editors
were Joseph J. Brehm and Bernice Heller.
Peter D. Guilmette supervised production.*

This investigation
was supported by the W. K. Kellogg Foundation
and the Avalon Foundation,
and by a private individual.

COMMISSIONERS

President of the Commission

W. ALLEN WALLIS
President
The University of Rochester
Rochester, New York

Vice President of the Commission

ROBERT K. MERTON, Ph.D.
Giddings Professor of Sociology
Department of Sociology
Columbia University
New York, New York

Secretary of the Commission

ELEANOR LAMBERTSEN, Ed.D.
Director
Division of Health Services, Sciences,
    and Education
Teachers College
Columbia University
New York, New York

RAY EVERETT BROWN
Executive Vice President
Northwestern University Medical Center
Chicago, Illinois

PREFACE

This volume is the report of the National Commission on Nursing and Nursing Education. The commission is unanimous in its findings and recommendations.

The report is based on two-and-a-half years' work by the commission and its staff. It reflects also the contributions of 34 members of four advisory panels and approximately 139 representatives of the health professions and of users of health services who reviewed preliminary materials at regional conferences or individually.

The commission held its first meeting on 19 September 1967 and its ninth and final meeting on 20 January 1970. We kept in close touch with our staff through 27 newsletters sent to us within the first two working days of each month. These described work in progress, completed, and planned, and sometimes were supplemented by exhibits. Staff members conferred from time to time with members of the commission by phone or by visit. Various drafts of the findings, the recommendations, and eventually the chapters of this report were sent to the commissioners for revision, and most of the final versions included in this report were approved in commission meetings. Obviously, however, each commissioner cannot be held responsible for each word and nuance.

On behalf of the commission I want to thank our Director, Jerome P. Lysaught, his Associate Director, Charles H. Russell, and their colleagues. They were unusual among the staffs of such commissions in keeping to their schedule, consulting widely, maintaining excellence in the work, and achieving complete articulation with the members of the commission.

It is a pleasure to acknowledge the financial support of the Avalon (now Mellon) and Kellogg Foundations and of an anonymous individual donor. To the American Nursing Association and the National League for Nursing, in particular to Inez Haynes and Judith Whitaker, who were then their executive directors, goes credit for organizing the commission, which was incorporated independently as a not-for-profit corporation, entirely controlled by the commissioners.

As President of the commission, I extend thanks to the other members. They left nothing to be desired in dedication, industry, competence, and conscientiousness. They were always congenial, even during the most vigorous debates. We enjoyed working together and we learned a lot from one another. We hope that our report will help improve health care for the American people.

W. Allen Wallis
The University of Rochester

2 April 1970

ACKNOWLEDGEMENTS

From the inception of this study, our staff has referred frequently to two earlier investigations of the health professions as guides, and as comparison rods, to the development of our own design and procedures. We gratefully acknowledge the help of Abraham Flexner's *Medical Education in the United States and Canada* and Esther Lucile Brown's *Nursing for the Future.*

Through our study of the Flexner report, we developed an appreciation for the acquisition of authenticated information through the comparison of report data and personal observations. We learned something of the process of distilling recommendations from large quantities of data, and projecting practical plans for implementation. With the benefit of 60 years' elapsed time, we also discovered the problems attendant on trying to obtain quality in professional education through a drastic reduction in the quantity of preparatory institutions.

Our debt to Dr. Brown is even greater. She provided us with remarkable insight into the investigatory field we were entering, and the resemblance between the two final methodologies is quite strong. We would not be loath to say that we copied our design from her if this were the case. Odd as it may seem, however, following an independent course, we kept finding, at each step, that our decisions basically replicated hers.

For example, we were initially instructed by the commission to determine how we could improve the delivery of health care to the American people through an analysis and improvement of nursing practice and nursing education. The first decision reached by Brown was "to view nursing service and nursing education in terms of what is best for society—not what is best for the profession of nursing."

Our study staff appointed two advisory groups in the first months of its existence with the consent of the commission. These included a panel of nurses and one of other health specialists. Sometime later, we involved the lay public in a series of regional meetings to aid us in examining our findings. In the case of Brown, she began her study with a Professional Advisory Committee of nurses and a Lay Advisory Committee, and later augmented these groups with a body of health administrators and physicians.

Both the present study and the Brown investigation made extensive use of site visitation, and both took pains to include regional variation and geographic distribution in the planning of these meetings. Dr. Brown visited some 50 schools of nursing; this study involved over 100 site visits to schools, hospitals, extended care facilities, and community health centers.

Both studies made use of regional conferences. The Brown study held three three-day conferences for directors of schools of nursing and for representatives of state boards of nursing, public health agencies, and other bodies that employed large nursing staffs. The current investigation held one round of regional meetings which included nurse educators, nurse practitioners, other health professionals, and public representatives. This was followed by a round of meetings with selected spokesmen for the major professional organizations, the ANA, NLN, AMA, and AHA. We then conducted a second series of regional meetings, 13 in all, to discuss the findings and plan for implementation. All these sessions in both studies were designed to broaden the base of participation.

A final point of comparison is embodied in Dr. Brown's statement that the answers to how nursing should be organized, administered, and financed had to be reached by a long, circuitous route. Like her, we found that the problems of nursing education could be answered only in light of projections concerning nursing roles and functions. Moreover, the questions of nursing careers could be approached only through an understanding of both educational patterns and requirements of practice. This did, indeed, involve a long, circuitous route, but it was absolutely impossible to dissect any one of these concerns without thought to its relationship to the other elements in the triad—nursing roles, nursing education, and nursing careers.

It has been a source of great encouragement to us that so many of these decisions and approaches bear a striking resemblance. At the same time, because this was an instance of an almost classic descriptive research design, coupled with direct and indirect analysis, one should expect basic similarity to related research.

In the period between October, 1967, and February, 1968, the core of the staff group developed the protocols for the research investigation The commissioners went over those research proposals quite intensively. Each one contributed valuable criticism and expertise. I know the other commissioners will not mind our singling out the contributions of three individuals from that group who made particular individual contributions to our thinking and design. Lowell Coggeshall, who was instrumental in the investigation of *Planning for Medical Progress Through Education,* could analyze our proposals from the vantage point of having conducted a most significant study of the medical profession. Ralph Tyler's contributions are myriad, but he particularly helped us through his development of indirect analysis techniques in his own research for the Air University. Robert Merton proffered his great wisdom in sociological inquiry and ensured that our use of Likert scales and other instruments was appropriate to the purpose intended.

It would be a case of gilding the lily to recount the contributions of the other commissioners. They were acute, incisive, and, though sometimes critical, always supportive. I would have 'to add, however, that our three nurse commissioners served double duty. They not only participated in each phase of the study along with the others, but they served as perpetual representatives of both commission and staff. They were required to explain, to interpret—and indeed to defend—the decisions, the methodology, and the work of the investigation. If the staff has developed a strong affection for Eleanor Lambertsen, Margaret Dolan, and Mary Jane McCarthy it is simply because they have been remarkable people.

Within the staff itself, Dr. Charles Russell has ably served as Associate Director and has personally directed the aspects of the inquiry into nursing careers. His experience with the earlier study on *Liberal Education and Nursing* proved a great asset to the entire staff. Raymond Burrows, initially, and Maryann Powers, subsequently, directed the inquiry into nursing roles and functions. Richard Huse has served in many capacities, but has borne primary responsibility for the development and analyses of the appendix material which will be separately published. Sydney Sutherland wondered at one time what the title Assistant to the Director encompassed. She learned that it meant seeing to everything that needed doing and helping everyone who needed aid. She did precisely that.

Our administrative and clerical staff aided us immeasurably even though individuals did depart at points along the way. Herman Kauz helped us to organize and develop our systems before he left to join the staff of the National League for Nursing. Judith Dorman Whitney served as our first, and, for a long period, only, secretary. She left us because she had her own contribution to make to our concerns over the population explosion. She and her husband just didn't seem to share our worry—neither did their bouncing son. Lois Patterson, Barbara DeRose, and Katherine Thompson have shared in the work, and we trust in the satisfaction, of seeing the report and the recommendations come to life under their fingers. Jill Orioli who ostensibly works at other projects in The University of Rochester spent so many evenings and lunch hours helping on rush projects that she has been adopted as a staff member—and deserves far better than that.

For that which is good and will become lasting in this inquiry, the staff and the commission have earned full recognition. For any errors of omission or commission, the director bears full responsibility. No research director ever had a more reinforcing group of "bosses"; no worker ever had a more self-directive, industrious body of associates. Together, staff and commission have labored to produce this report. We are content to let the document and the recommendations speak for themselves. Our greatest hope is that it will receive a full hearing from the professions and the public—who are the ones the whole thing is about.

Jerome P. Lysaught
Director

17 March 1970

STUDY STAFF

DR. JEROME P. LYSAUGHT
Director

DR. CHARLES H. RUSSELL
Associate Director

MISS SYDNEY ANNE SUTHERLAND
Assistant to the Director

MR. RAYMOND BURROWS
Research Associate

MR. RICHARD E. HUSE
Research Associate

MISS MARYANN E. POWERS
Research Associate

MR. HERMAN KAUZ
Staff Administrator

MISS GILDA M. ORIOLI
Secretary

MRS. JUDITH D. WHITNEY
Secretary

CONTENTS

Commissioners   vii
Preface   ix
Acknowledgements   xi
Study Staff   xv

Chapter 1   ORIGIN, OBJECTIVES, AND METHODS OF THIS
             INVESTIGATION   1

    Composition of the commission   2
    Appointment of a study staff   3
    Timetable for the study   3
    Delineation of Key Problems   4
    Supply and demand for nurses   4
    Nursing roles and functions   5
    Nursing education   6
    Nursing careers   6
    A composite of situations   7
    The Trends in Health Care and Delivery   7
    Social and cultural changes   8
    Advances in medical science   9

Changed economics of health   9
Summary of emerging trends   11
Objectives of the Study   11
Roles and functions   12
Nursing education   12
Nursing careers   13
Methods of the Study   14
Nursing advisory panel   15
Health professions advisory panel   16
Literature search and surveys   16
Site visits   18
Invitational conferences and meetings   18
Prospects for Change   21
Summary   23
Footnotes   23

Chapter 2   NURSING IN THE AMERICAN HEALTH SCENE   25

Nursing and the Nation's Health   26
Historical Development of Professional Nursing   28
Current Problems and Trends in Nursing   32
Level of commitment   33
Long and disciplined educational process   35
Unique body of knowledge and skill   38
Discretionary authority and judgment   40
Active and cohesive professional organization   41
Summary   44
Footnotes   45

Chapter 3   THE CHARACTERISTICS, CONCEPTS, AND SCOPE
             OF NURSING PRACTICE   49

Characteristics of Nursing Practice   49
Climate of nursing shortage   50
Climate of impoverished work environment   53
Climate of role misunderstanding   56
Summary of nursing climate   58
Concepts of Nursing Practice   58
The public image of nursing   58
The occupational view of nursing   60
Nursing as an emerging professional practice   62

Impact of the rival perceptions   64
Scope of Nursing Practice   64
A model of nursing practice   64
The changing scope of nursing practice   69
Effects of nursing practice   73
Summary   75
Footnotes   76

Chapter 4   FINDINGS AND RECOMMENDATIONS ON
                   NURSING ROLES AND FUNCTIONS   81

Research into Nursing Practice   83
Role Articulation in Health Practice   87
Organization of Nursing Roles   90
Leadership for Nursing Practice   94
Technology and Changing Systems   96
Footnotes   98

Chapter 5   FINDINGS AND RECOMMENDATIONS ON
                   NURSING EDUCATION   101

Institutional Patterns for Nursing Education   103
Problems of Preparatory Institutions   110
Accreditation of Educational Institutions   113
Curricular Needs and Articulation   114
Graduate Study and Faculty Development   117
Institutional Admission and Retention   120
Continuing and In-Service Education   122
Financing of the Recommendations   123
Footnotes   127

Chapter 6   FINDINGS AND RECOMMENDATIONS ON
                   NURSING CAREERS   129

Planning for Nursing Careers   130
Retention of Qualified Practitioners   132
Recruitment of Nursing Students   136
New sources of manpower supply   137

Licensure and Career Performance   141

Professional Organization and Nursing Leadership   144

Footnotes   146

Chapter 7   SUMMARY AND CONCLUSIONS   149

Reflections Concerning This Study   149

Limitations of the Study   151

Focus of the Study   153

Atmosphere of the Study   154

A Summary of the Results   154

An Abstract for Action   161

Conclusion   163

Footnotes   164

GLOSSARY OF TERMS   165

AN ABSTRACT FOR ACTION

ONE
ORIGIN, OBJECTIVES, AND METHODS OF THIS INVESTIGATION

The impetus for this study of nursing and nursing education can be traced directly to the 1963 report of the Surgeon General's Consultant Group on Nursing. In their final document, *Toward Quality in Nursing*,[1] those experts recommended a national investigation of nursing education with special emphasis on the responsibilities and skills required for high-quality patient care. While the group endorsed the provision of funds for such a study, it had completed its own work and could not offer direct financial assistance.

Shortly after this report appeared, the two major organizations in nursing—the American Nurses' Association and the National League for Nursing—appropriated funds and established a joint committee to study the ways to conduct and finance such a national inquiry. After much exploration this committee decided that there was a need to examine not only the changing practices and educational patterns in nursing today but also the probable requirements in professional nursing over the next several decades. In April of 1966, W. Allen Wallis, President of The University of Rochester, agreed to head such a study if adequate financing could be obtained.

While few questioned the desirability of a national study of nursing, many foundations and government agencies had reservations over the timing of the investigation because the President's National Advisory Commission on Health Manpower was preparing to examine the manpower requirements of all the health professions. However, the Board of Directors of the American Nurses' Foundation— confident that the problems in nursing were far more wide-ranging than the matter of manpower—voted in the fall of 1966 to grant up to $50,000 to help launch the present study. This willingness to back up conviction with capital played a key role in the decisions by the Avalon Foundation and the Kellogg Foundation to grant $100,000 each to support this investigation. Coincidentally, an anonymous bene-factor contributed the sum of $300,000 to ensure the undertaking.

On January 5, 1967, the members of the joint committee met with Mr. Wallis to discuss the organization and membership of the commission as well as the ap-pointment of a study director.

This brief summary is intended not only to serve as an overview of the pre-liminary timetable for the investigation, but also to underline a key facet of the structure of support for the study. While the commission was a direct outgrowth of the keen interest of the ANA and NLN, it was set up as an independent agency and functioned as a self-directing group, with the power to plan and conduct its in-vestigations as it saw fit.

Such freedom of action demanded responsibility of leadership, and Mr. Wallis emphasized that no commissioner should be selected to represent an interest group or a particular position. Rather, the commissioners should be chosen for their broad knowledge of nursing; for their skills in related disciplines like medicine and health administration; or for their competencies in relevant fields like economics, education, management, and social research. The commissioners should represent individual excellence and collective mastery of a host of special-ized areas that are interwoven with the major challenges facing nursing today.

Composition of the Commission

It was no easy task to determine which individuals should be asked to serve and then to approach these busy people with our request for their time and commit-ment for a major project. In August, 1967, the first meeting of the newly appointed commissioners took place, and only some time later did we reach the full com-plement of 12. At that initial session, however, the incorporating members from the joint committee resigned and the destiny of the study was placed in the hands of the independent commission, whose members are the following:

> Ray Everett Brown, Executive Vice President of the Northwestern University Medi-cal Center (over much of the course of this study, he served as Executive Vice Presi-dent of the Affiliated Hospital Center, Boston).
> Lowell T. Coggeshall, M.D., Former Assistant to the Secretary of Health, Education, and Welfare.

Margaret B. Dolan, Head of Department of Public Health Nursing, School of Public Health, University of North Carolina.

Marion B. Folsom, Former Secretary of Health, Education, and Welfare.

Walter E. Hoadley, Ph.D., Executive Vice President, Bank of America National Trust and Savings Association.

Eleanor Lambertsen, Ed.D., Director of Division of Health Services, Sciences and Education, Teachers College, Columbia University.

Herbert E. Longenecker, Ph.D., President, Tulane University.

Mary Jane McCarthy, Director, Nursing Service, Veterans Administration.

Leonard F. McCollum, Chairman of the Board, Continental Oil Company.

Robert K. Merton, Ph.D., Giddings Professor of Sociology, Columbia University.

Ralph W. Tyler, Ph.D., Former Director, Center for Advanced Study in Behavioral Sciences, Palo Alto.

W. Allen Wallis, President, The University of Rochester.

In addition to their service as commissioners, Mr. Wallis functioned as President, Mr. Merton as Vice President, and Miss Lambertsen as Secretary. The Treasurer and Assistant Treasurer, LaRoy B. Thompson and Kenneth E. Wood, held the responsibilities of these offices, but were not members of the commission and did not take part in its deliberations.

Appointment of a Study Staff

At the first formal meeting of the commission, in August of 1967, a director, Dr. Jerome P. Lysaught, and an associate director, Dr. Charles H. Russell, were appointed to conduct the planning and actual operation of the inquiry. A headquarters was established in Rochester, New York, through the cooperation of the university, and a small staff was acquired to develop the research proposal. Subsequently, additional individuals were drawn in, on either a full- or part-time basis, to carry out the provisions of the protocols.* The staff members were able to do some planning in December, 1967, but the project became truly operational in January of 1968, and its timetable was predicated from that point on.

Timetable for the Study

The original proposal for the investigation provided for a three-year study of nursing and nursing education. In the specific plan developed by the study staff, a number of interim deadlines were established, and an overall goal of three years was set, dating from the first session of the commissioners and the appointment of the directors. This meant that the general objectives should be reached by Septem-

*A listing and acknowledgement of the contribution of the individuals on the study staff is provided in the *Acknowledgements* to the full report.

ber, 1970. As a result, the final report and recommendations were due by the end of January, 1970, so that several months would be available for follow-up activities. These would include information meetings, dissemination of the recommendations, and staff appearances before groups vital to the enactment of any proposed changes. In addition, our planning included the provision for a contingency operation of up to three full years from the start of the study (until January, 1971) so that we could initiate the implementation of the recommendations — a beginning effort we felt would be vital to the project.

DELINEATION OF KEY PROBLEMS

The major preparation and funding invested in this nationwide study presupposed the obvious fact that we would find essential problems in American nursing that needed to be solved. On this point there was no disagreement. After the Second World War, deep-seated conflicts had accumulated within the profession itself, and more particularly, between nursing and the other two members of the traditional health triangle, medicine and administration. Some of these disagreements had surfaced until they were publicly recognized; others were played out within the confines of the individual organizations and health facilities. But underlying all these problems were deeper ones that stemmed from the essential fabric of health care in the United States today. Four of these require particular attention.

Supply and Demand for Nurses

It is a safe assumption that any discussion of health manpower during the past 25 years has occasioned a lament over the lack of nurses. Newspapers have reported critical shortages of nurses in hospitals, and even the closing of wards and services. Projections by a number of data gathering agencies have predicted a shortage of hundreds of thousands of nurses by 1975, and have generally suggested that the situation will get worse, not better. In this climate, it was inevitable that the public and the press voice a widespread demand for training more nurses and preparing thousands of additional aides and auxiliaries.

Occasionally, a voice was heard to suggest that the problem might be one of misuse rather than shortage. Or, to put it another way, that improving the economic and social satisfactions of nursing might quickly relieve the shortage of nurses by returning to the manpower pool some of the hundreds of thousands of individuals who had retired from active careers. Still other observers, mostly economists, argued that the proposed solutions for adding thousands of nurses and nurse aides would have the opposite effect, namely, more nurses would further depress salaries and result in a still greater flight from professional activity.

The man on the street is to be excused if his reaction to these rival claims is one of confusion and doubt. Is there indeed a nursing shortage? And, if so, how is it to be solved? One thing is certain. It is crucial that we adopt an independent, nondoctrinaire approach in determining the nature and extent of the problems and what might reasonably be done to change the system.

Nursing Roles and Functions

Because of the rising demands for health service, and because there are critical shortages among physicians as well as nurses, there have been many suggestions for basic reorganization of the nursing role. More and more, the term "physician's assistant" has been brought into play. From the standpoint of many, it makes sense to have the nurse take over as many functions from the doctor as she can capably handle. A number of states have taken steps to change medical practice laws that restrict the nurse from engaging in activities that are performed traditionally by physicians. At the same time, however, the current controversy over nurses acting as anesthetists or midwives illustrates the confusion in both medicine and nursing over the functions and limitations of nursing practice. Even the natural evolution of health and educational institutions has seemed to draw nurses away from the bedside and into higher paying posts as administrators and educators—but not as patient care specialists. Finally, the nurse remaining on the ward has found herself essentially "nursing through others," directing the activities of nurse aides and assistants while frequently performing the necessary, though hardly related, tasks of supervising housecleaning, assessing patient charges, training nonprofessional employees, and ordering supplies.

In contrast to these developments, the professional nursing organizations were becoming more aware of internal shifts in their members' views. A growing number of nurses were quite vocal in their demand for increased emphasis on clinical practice. Higher education programs that led to positions in administration and teaching were declared less relevant than newly established concentrations in a clinical specialty. Nurses cooperated with physicians in developing higher levels of treatment and intervention, but were adamant in maintaining a distinction between nursing and medical practice.

A further enigma lay in the impact of increased technology. At one stroke, these advancements made some traditional procedures obsolete while creating wholly new health specialties. The computer might take over all sorts of record-keeping, but transplant operations required technicians and teams that had never been provided before in the organization plans of hospitals and operating rooms.

No one had ready answers for such questions as these: What is the best organization or reorganization of institutions, disciplines, and roles to meet current and future health care needs? What is the role of the nurse today? In the decades ahead? How can we set up mechanisms for continuing change in the face of tradition and social lag? These are the crucial concerns that require independent analysis, utilizing the best input from nursing and the other health professions — as well as the viewpoint of the patient, the eventual consumer of all health care.

Nursing Education

The problems within the institutions for educating nurses are quite as great as those facing the individual practitioner. They have been made even more spectacular by the heat of controversy that has raged about them. There has been a significant shift over the past 25 years in the programs for preparing nurses. At one time, hospital schools prepared almost all professional nurses. These nurses received a diploma on graduation, and the R.N. license upon successful completion of examination. For a combination of reasons, some obvious, others less evident, almost 50 percent of the hospital schools have closed in recent years. The number of nursing graduates has grown, but largely as the result of newly established nursing programs in colleges and junior colleges.

The professional organization of nurses, the American Nurses' Association, has gone on record with the resolution that all nursing education should be housed in institutions of higher education; the remaining hospital schools should be phased out according to a definite plan. However, many nurses, and even more physicians and administrators, feel that there is much to commend the hospital school approach with its built-in emphasis on patient care and clinical experience. Once this issue was joined, emotions became intensified and organizational positions hardened.

At the same time, the public is asking some elemental questions that must be answered: What are the best institutions for producing nurses? Which institutions will attract the kinds of students that nursing needs? And what should be the course of study for these students? All these questions are essential and must be examined apart from partisan proclamation or organizational pronouncement.

Nursing Careers

Interwoven among all the preceding considerations are problems of retaining nurses in active careers. At any given time, one of three professional nurses is inactive. In great part, this is because nursing is a woman's profession. Childbearing and family-rearing take their toll in the length of women's working lives. But the causes would seem to be more complex than this. Is there anything that can develop a greater commitment to the pursuit of a career? Should nursing overtly attempt to discard its feminine image and seek to attract a dramatically larger proportion of men into its ranks?

A Composite of Situations

It is tempting to deal separately with these four key problems of nursing and to isolate them from the overall pattern of health care in the United States. As a consequence, we have seen vigorous efforts to educate and graduate more nurses in order to *solve* the nursing problem. To an extent, this has been successful. Certainly the nursing profession has kept pace with, and even exceeded, the growth of population. Yet, we still find shortages. Can the real cause stem from our failure to recognize the problems in the nursing role that siphon away so many professionals? Is it because there is a whole new universe of needs for nurses? Is it also because we have failed to organize and articulate the educational process so that meaningful career opportunities are available to each individual? Is the training of the student relevant to the ultimate demands she will face? And, finally, is the current shortage related, in part, to the discouraging turnover among nursing personnel, and to the great body of inactive nurses who find the rewards of their profession less attractive than alternative pursuits?

In our effort to provide an independent look at nursing and to suggest solutions for its problems, we have found it necessary to examine not only the nature of its key concerns but also to relate these issues to the social system that provides the entire spectrum of health care for the American public.

THE TRENDS IN HEALTH CARE AND DELIVERY

As the *Report of the National Advisory Commission on Health Manpower* puts it so succinctly, "There *is* a crisis in American health care."[2] Nor is such an observation reserved to the occasional report or monograph. The popular press has fastened on the faults of the health care system and has blazoned articles on its costs, its impersonality, and its less-than-adequate delivery systems for portions of the population. Further, these unfavorable observations are substantiated not only by the acknowledgement of the American Nurses' Association but also by the reasoned criticism of the American Medical Association and numerous other voices among the practitioners and respected medical educators. Similarly the American Hospital Association, the Blue Cross plans, and other major organizations have admitted to deficiencies and oversights in planning and care.

This, in turn, would seem to raise the greatest paradox in our social history. Is it possible that the American health system can reputedly be the finest in the world, as many contend, and still be guilty of the faults that its critics claim? The simplest and most honest answer may be Yes. The very system that has contributed so mightily to the conquest of disease has not been able to distribute the fruits of its research equally to those in need. The same nation that has attempted to export medicine and knowledge to combat plague and infection throughout much of the world is now importing doctors and nurses from countries that can least afford to see them go. The health services that have served as frequent models for nations developing new schools of medicine and nursing are now unable to produce the numbers of graduates that their own professional societies report as minimum to provide reasonable health care throughout the country.

The awareness of these shortcomings, and indeed the existence of many of them, come as a direct result of several forces that have appeared over the past 25 years. Any attempt at the solution of health care problems, and the problems of nursing in particular, must take into account the following trends.

Social and Cultural Changes

The United States has recognized the existence of a population explosion since the Second World War. Overcrowded schools, increased taxes to underwrite municipal and suburban growth, and problems of traffic, congestion, and pollution are all aspects of our gigantic population growth. Moreover, the United States continues to have a higher marriage rate and a lower age for entering marriage than most other industrial countries. The inevitable result: more crowding and worse problems.

From the standpoint of the health care system, there is a second facet to the dilemma. The very success of medical research and individual care, coupled, of course, with better diets, housing, and general living conditions, has produced a dramatic increase in life expectancy over the last three generations. More people are living longer and, consequently, requiring more long-term care than we have ever been called on to provide before.

Essentially, the health system is facing a rising bimodal needs curve that represents the very young and the very old—both groups requiring more care and more dependence on the health practitioner.

The increased urbanization that has accompanied our population growth, signaled by the development of the megalopolis, has further aggravated the problems of health care. Rural areas are sometimes depleted of health professionals. Because of shifts in residential patterns, many urban institutions and health care facilities are no longer in population centers; in other cases, these facilities were never designed to meet the needs of the changed community, and therefore are not equipped to serve the ill and the injured. In contrast, advances in communication have made it possible to herald new discoveries and treatments in health care more rapidly than ever before. Thus, the public is more fully aware of the potentials than the problems of the health professions. The electronic world of McCluhan has outstripped our twentieth century ability to translate the possibility into the reality.

Advances in Medical Science

Less tangible to us, but quite as important as our population growth, are the advancements in the biological and medical sciences. In our lifetime, we have seen dread diseases effectively controlled, if not eliminated. We have looked on with astonishment as recipients of transplants and artificial organs have resumed almost normal living patterns. Similar advances in psychiatric treatment and in mental and public health have encouraged the hope that unborn generations may live in freedom from the ravages of disease and pestilence and emotional disorder that we have known.

These events, as with increased life expectancy, have multiple effects on the health system as well as on the individuals who benefit from treatment. New specialties must rise; new institutions must be erected; and new organizations must be developed to translate laboratory breakthroughs into operational realities as the world enters the twenty-first century.

Advances in medical science are not necessarily accompanied by improvements in distribution. Many hundreds of health facilities, and thousands of chronic care institutions, have been built since the Second World War. Few of them are planned, equipped, and manned so that they can readily adjust to the ever-changing conditions of medical science or society. In the same way, professional practitioners, including nurses, have not reacted quickly to the changing demands of their roles. In this they are not alone; but the public may soon begin to clamor for improved conditions. When there is no real hope for change, people can be tolerant. When hope is aroused through medical advancement and the communications media, then the public becomes intolerant of the impediments that stand in the way of new services, especially when such impediments stem from inertia, tradition, or inability to change old habits among health care professions and institutions.

Changed Economics of Health

A greater population base and exciting new developments in medicine, in themselves, would not generate public demand for drugs and treatment unless people had the funds available to pay for these services. Thus, we see that, along with increased population and technological advancements, significant changes have been brought about in our system of paying medical costs.

Our population as a whole is rising to new levels of income and education. This situation produces individuals who are more knowledgeable about health care, more concerned about obtaining professional medical services, and better able to pay the bills that result. An even more revolutionary force, however, is the growth of prepaid medical and surgical insurance plans, supplemented in part by governmental programs for Medicare and Medicaid. Today, patients are not only better able to afford medical costs, but increasing numbers, through insurance, prepayment plans and government programs, now have almost unlimited access to the finest health care resources that are available to them. The result is a tremendous increase in the call for health professionals and more extensive use of all health care facilities.

At the same time, there is growing social awareness of the inequities in the distribution of our health care resources. Forces are at work to extend the domain of insurance and governmental aid to include population groups without adequate coverage and to enlarge and coordinate the planned attack on such maladies as heart disease, cancer, and stroke. Regional and national programs have been developed to supplement the local and state agencies that have, in the past, attempted to cope with problems of disease.

Experience has taught us that providing health insurance to large bodies of population without parallel increases in facilities and health personnel can lead to chaotic consequences. Yet, the current advocates of national health insurance have not always looked beyond their primary objective to examine the crucial need for increasing the number of physicians, nurses, and facilities to accommodate the enlarged demand. Human beings exist in a real world; performance must somehow square with promises. Today, the rise in our national income, and in the percentage that we can use for health services, has already threatened to overwhelm our health industry. With more than three-fourths of our population now covered by health insurance, and with the possibility that this figure may soon be close to 100 percent, our ability to live up to our implied promises seems remote, at best.[3]

In addition, although the public has enjoyed greater income, it has also encountered steep rises in the price of health care. Consumer costs for health services have frequently risen more sharply than the general increase in prices. In the nine-year period from 1959 to 1968, for example, the cost of living rose 20 per cent; medical costs rose 45 percent; hospital costs soared 122 percent.[4]

Likewise, this upward trend is reflected in the costs of professional health education. The tuition charges have increased in most institutions preparing physicians and nurses. Schools and hospitals encounter rising construction costs when they must enlarge their facilities or build new ones. In short, health is a big business enterprise that involves billions of dollars annually. Moreover, the expenditures for health care have grown at a logarithmic rate for years and show no signs of slowing down. Currently, the costs of health care account for more than 6 percent of the annual expenditures made by Americans, and the trend seems firmly established on an upward path.

Summary of Emerging Trends

These, then, are the facts of life within which our health care system must operate. If this system has failed to provide the kind of care that we would like, it is in large part because our population has grown enormously, and in ways that foster increased demands for greater care. At the same time, we are still groping for the institutions, facilities, and personal resources that can meet the public's demands and match the advances that have come through medical research.

In many ways, the public is just as responsible as the health industry for the lag in health care advances. Our ideal of the physician is still the general practitioner—the family doctor—at a time when we ask for services that demand the quintessence of specialization. We revere the personal identification of ourselves with "our doctor" when group practice and team performance in all phases of health care may be essential for quality care. We still seek a stereotype for our health care institutions when technology makes possible the automation of a facility for real advances in patient treatment.

If the public reaction to the situation described in the preceding paragraph is one of shock, it may be necessary to point out once again that industrial, social, electronic, and biomedical revolutions are already underway within our health care system. As these changing patterns broaden health care opportunities, so they increase its problems. No one wants depersonalized care. At the same time, no one should forego optimum care because of reverence for the conventional or the traditional. Thus, the central problem for all health professionals becomes how to control and implement change—how to incorporate today's advances with the still-useful practices of yesterday. It may be that nursing, in particular, holds the key to maintenance of humane, individualistic concern for people and their health problems. And this capacity must be zealously enlarged.

OBJECTIVES OF THE STUDY

Until now, in this report, we have been focusing on the emerging trends that affect our entire health system. At this point it is essential that we specify the primary objective of the investigation. Simply put, it is this: How can we improve the delivery of health care to the American people, particularly through the analysis and improvement of nursing and nursing education. People, as individuals, are the subjects and objects of health care. Care is required wherever people are gathered —in hospitals, clinics, nursing homes, factories. This is the *raison d'être* for nurses and nursing. Our efforts to enhance nursing and to improve the education, roles, and careers of nurses begin with the critical need to ensure that better health care is provided for the person who requires it.

If this seems a self-evident statement, let us underline the fact that the commission, as an independent body, is not seeking to ameliorate the lot of nurses as an end in itself. The commission is not interested in demarcating professional boundaries, except as these boundaries can contribute to a positive improvement in health care available to the American public. And it is this single criterion, better patient care for all people, that has served as the measuring rod for the findings and recommendations in this report.

Given this imperative, there are three areas into which the study can be divided: nursing roles and functions; nursing education; and nursing careers.

Roles and Functions

In the area of nursing practice, traditional role expectations are being challenged by changes in health care and in the institutions that provide it. The influences of advanced technology and new specializations are being felt already. Nevertheless, the conventional patterns of nursing utilization still determine individual assignments, status, manpower, and job satisfaction. Our goals in studying this area have been the following:

a. To improve definitions of patient-care functions and activities for more effective utilization of nurses.

b. To identify needs, institutions, and organizational patterns that will have major impact on changing nurse roles.

c. To identify new resources, staffing patterns, and methods of distribution through which quality nursing care can be extended and improved.

d. To examine innovative settings and professional relationships which suggest emerging role differentiation, and project the impact of these on future health care.

In brief, this portion of the investigation was aimed at anticipating and predicting changing role requirements so that nurses could be utilized more effectively and quality care could be extended in a rapidly changing health system.

Nursing Education

An incongruous feature of nursing education today stems from the wide variety of programs that lead to licensure as a registered nurse. Students who have studied for one and one-half, two, three, four, or even five years are accorded the same license, which is accompanied by a diploma, an associate degree, a bachelor degree, or even a graduate degree.

Concerns about nursing education go far deeper than the variants in prepara- tory training, however. Another crucial consideration is the relationship between the nurse educator and the nurse practitioner—and the institutions that house them. How closely meshed are learning and practice? How aware are teachers of innovative practice? How versed are practitioners in the developments from re- search? And what about the institutions for educating nurses? There are 1,300 preparatory nursing programs in the United States. How many possess adequate faculty, resources, and funding to provide quality education? In examining these and related issues, there were fundamental questions to be answered:

a. How can the institutions for nursing education be assessed? What are their resources, their needs, and their objectives?

b. Who are the students? Where do they come from? Are there untapped sources for providing more quality students?

c. Who are the individuals on the faculty? What are their capabilities, their needs?

d. What about the nursing curriculum? Is it fixed or changing? Does it relate to innovations in research and practice? Is it generalized or individualized? How much experimentation is taking place? Is there variety among institutions?

e. What are the opportunities for continuing education? What about educational choices that can complement career ladders? Who is responsible for the quality of in-service education?

By developing data on these areas, we felt that we could understand both the current and projected problems among nursing schools and recommend mea- sures to anticipate the pressures that will face students, faculty, and institutions in the years ahead.

Nursing Careers

To gain insight into the disputed area of manpower requirements, and to understand the reasons for high rates of inactivity among nurse graduates, we investigated the career opportunities and satisfactions of these individuals. While we undertook a wide-ranging inquiry in this area, a few of our questions might suggest the variety of concerns that we explored:

a. What will be the future *need* and *demand* for nurses in the face of trends toward increased population, urbanization, and calls for health care?

b. What steps can be taken to retain graduates in active pursuit of professional nursing?

c. What effect will the trends toward masterly clinical performance have on career goals? Will they enhance or retard longer work patterns?

d. What are the emerging relationships between nursing and medicine? Between nursing and other health professions? How can these be improved?

e. What are the legal implications of changing patterns? What of licensure and specialty recognition?

Clearly, nursing needs interdisciplinary approaches and cooperative study with other professions to determine current data, emerging directions, and needed changes. From these findings, recommendations could be developed to improve patient care through enhanced career opportunities in nursing.

METHODS OF THE STUDY

To attain the objectives of the study, we decided that two general approaches were necessary: the analysis of current practices and patterns, and the assessment of future needs. To state it simply, we hoped to take the best from what is available today and develop ways to enhance direct patient care for tomorrow. This meant that at the outset our investigation consisted of many observational and descriptive tasks, combined with the collection and analysis of the findings from other studies. In succeeding phases of the project, we subjected our findings and recommendations, plus our projections for the future, to the scrutiny of a great number of groups and individuals involved in the delivery of health care. From their comments, suggestions, and criticisms we attempted to substantiate both the authenticity of our observations and the validity of our projections.

The approach of observation and accumulation of baseline data, followed by analysis of both external forces and internal pressures, resulting in formulation of recommendations for change, is a common one in the behavioral sciences and certainly not unique to this study. In our case, it is consciously patterned after Flexner's inquiry into American medicine and refined by the experience of other professional studies that have been conducted in the last quarter century.

The quality of such a study and its accuracy are largely determined by the willingness of the investigators to admit not only a full range of data into their analyses, but also to invoke the interpretations of specialists from many points of view. In this investigation we have tried to make sure that rival interpretations and alternative proposals for change are given as full consideration as possible.

Nursing Advisory Panel

Very early in the development of our study proposal, the staff and commission agreed that a permanent advisory panel of nurses would be a valuable resource. Such a body would advise on the plans for the study, suggest locations and sites for visitation, and generally review and criticize each stage of our work. The individual members of the panel were selected by the staff, in consultation with the commission and through a preliminary survey of the literature that served to identify many of the leaders in the nursing profession. The particular advisors who were chosen and who agreed to participate represented highly individual capacities to contribute to the various objectives of the study. They were not asked to represent organizational or institutional points of view, but *in toto,* they displayed a varied background of nursing service, and included individuals associated with all the current preparatory programs in nursing education. The panel was composed of these individuals:

Myrtle K. Aydelotte, Ph.D., Director, Department of Nursing Service, The University of Iowa.

Jeanne Berthold, Ph.D., Professor, Frances Payne Bolton School of Nursing, Case Western Reserve University.

Luther Christman, Ph.D., Dean, School of Nursing, Vanderbilt University.

Margaret E. Courtney, Ph.D., Associate Director, The Johns Hopkins School of Nursing.

Ellen Fahy, Ed.D., Dean, School of Nursing, State University of New York at Stony Brook, Health Sciences Center.

Katherine D. Foster, Former Director of Nursing, The University of Connecticut Health Center, presently Nurse Coordinator, Boston Maternal and Infant, Children and Youth Program.

Sister Virginia Kingsbury, Former Nursing Education Consultant, Daughters of Charity of St. Vincent DePaul.

Beatrice Perlmutter, Ed.D., Head, Department of Nursing, Bronx Community College of the City of New York.

Doris E. Roberts, Ph.D., Chief, Community Nursing Branch, Division of Nursing, Department of Health, Education, and Welfare.

Kathryn Smith, Ed.D., Dean and Professor, School of Nursing, University of Colorado.

Both individually and collectively, these panelists have examined succeeding drafts of our findings and recommendations. Their diversity of background and concern has been invaluable in our effort to gain understanding of the different interpretations that surround the essential trends in nursing practice and education today.

Health Professions Advisory Panel

Just as we sought diversity in the nurse advisory panel, so the staff and commission felt that we must have input from other individuals who would be profoundly affected by decisions about nursing. In this case, we asked individuals to serve on a health professions advisory panel—not to represent organizational or institutional points of view, but to ensure that each finding and recommendation was scrutinized by a group of people with a broad background of experience and understanding. The advisory panelists were these:

> Stuart H. Altman, Ph.D., Associate Professor of Economics, Brown University.
> Barbara Bates, M.D., Associate Professor of Medicine, The University of Rochester.
> Charles E. Berry, Associate Dean, School of Nursing, St. Louis University.
> Ivan J. Fahs, Ph.D., Upper Midwest Nursing Study, Minneapolis.
> Robert J. Haggerty, M.D., Professor of Pediatrics, The University of Rochester.
> Edmund D. Pellegrino, M.D., Vice President for the Health Sciences, State University of New York at Stony Brook.
> William Ruhe, M.D., Secretary, Council on Medical Education, American Medical Association.
> Daniel Schechter, Assistant to the Director, American Hospital Association.
> William K. Selden, Ph.D., Director, Commonwealth of Virginia, Governor's Committee on Nursing.
> Peter Terenzio, Executive Vice President, The Roosevelt Hospital.

The comments of this panel were invaluable in ensuring that a well-rounded analysis was made of each content area developed in the study. In addition, the two advisory groups provided us with a means for determining consensus and reasonable compromise in terms of the needs of the health field and the rival proposals that had been advanced for solving the most pressing problems. The contributions of these two panels cannot be overestimated in the improvement of all recommendations formulated by the study staff.

Literature Search and Surveys

After the appointment of the advisory panels, the staff began the task of sorting through the data contained in the literature along with the development of specific surveys to obtain missing information. We examined a sample of national and international publications, issue by issue, for the preceding three years. Moreover, a general literature search was conducted of all articles and research reports on nursing practice, nursing education, and nursing careers.

The references in those articles were used to uncover large quantities of unpublished reports. This effort was supplemented, with the active cooperation of the U.S. Public Health Service and other agencies, by the scanning of research abstracts and reports that had been funded in whole or in part by government grants. These thousands of items were finally reduced to some 900 bibliographic citations that seemed to bear heavily on our objectives. This number was subjected to further critical reading and review. When duplication and quality standards were invoked, the staff had annotated and organized more than 500 references produced in the preceding three years that were relevant to our project. In addition to creating a data retrieval bank this monumental task served as a valuable "basic course" to familiarize the entire staff with recent developments in nursing and the health care field.

We were aware of the existence of many state, regional, and national investigations into nursing or its subsidiary concerns in addition to the survey of current literature. To distill these findings and to ensure our consideration of historic developments, the staff compiled a thesaurus of these studies, collating and cross-referencing them so that results and recommendations could be seen clearly along a time line. Approximately 45 state and regional studies, completed within the preceding five years, were included along with ten national investigations into other health-related professions. Moreover, 15 national studies of nursing, either education or practice or both, were processed to give us a comprehensive picture of the relevant findings and recommendations from 1923 to the present.

The staff developed questionnaires and survey forms as well. The dean or director of each nursing preparatory program in the United States was questioned to determine the priority of problems facing nursing education. At the same time, we undertook a parallel survey with the heads of harboring institutions. We wanted to find out to what extent nursing's challenges were unique or were simply part and parcel of the problems involved in all phases of postsecondary education.

Likewise, the staff canvassed the institutions that had closed their nursing preparatory programs within the previous five years to find out their reasons for doing so, and to see if they had plans for resuming nursing education under new arrangements.

Two questionnaires were developed and distributed to nursing faculty and students selected through a randomized, stratified procedure. About 5,000 faculty members were asked to describe their activities, preparatory education, and background experience in nursing. More than 10,000 faculty members and students were asked to complete a Nursing Schools Environment Inventory (based on the Medical School Environment Inventory developed for the Association of American Medical Colleges). Through this extensive survey, we hoped to determine the attitudes and perceptions of future nurses about their education and to find out if there was a significant correlation between the student responses and the type of institution they attended. Similarly, we asked faculty members to react to the educational environment so that we could compare and contrast their answers with those of the students.

We distributed a booklet describing our preliminary findings to samples of nursing schools, directors of nursing services, state leagues for nursing, state nurse associations, state medical societies, and state hospital associations, along with many other groups and individuals, in order to disseminate our initial data and obtain further reactions and comments.

Finally, a number of short, specific questionnaires were addressed to such groups as state boards of nursing to obtain or verify information as the study progressed.

Site Visits

To supplement our review of the literature and results from the questionnaires, we planned a series of site visits to (a) examine institutions and practices that were widely recognized as outstanding, and (b) observe innovative practices and organizations that seemed to provide promising approaches for improving patient care.

No less than 143 sites were initially selected for inclusion in the study. After the staff had contacted these institutions, however, a total of 22 were dropped because of redundancy. The administrators of 20 other programs were able to supply complete reports that made a personal visit unnecessary. Thus, 100 site visits were made and in the process more than 1,000 individuals were interviewed. Among the varieties of activities that the staff observed were innovations in nursing education, curriculum experiments, innovative methods for utilizing nurse practitioners, and automated hospital environments.

Invitational Conferences and Meetings

As information was collected, the staff developed a preliminary set of indicated findings that could suggest directions for later recommendations. In addition to gaining the reactions of our advisory panels to these materials, we decided that an even wider exposure would be useful to ensure the balance and validity of our study. To accomplish this, we arranged for invitational regional conferences to be held in San Francisco, St. Louis, and Washington, D. C. We invited leaders in nursing service, nursing education, medicine, health administration, consumer groups, and third party payers to these meetings. Approximately 45 persons attended each meeting and participated in small-group discussions limited to 15 people.

The participants were asked to complete a Likert-scale reaction sheet on each finding and to make additional comments as they wished. Based on these responses, the staff then explored the need for additional study and modifications in the initial recommendations.

After the development of a second draft of possible recommendations, a series of small-group meetings was held with individuals from the American Nurses' Association, the National League for Nursing, the American Medical Association, the American Hospital Association, and others. These sessions involved their direct participation in discussing the recommendations, data base, effects, and possible alternatives. This pattern of communication provided criticism, understanding, and unique opportunities for developing consensus. Among the individuals who participated in this phase of our activities were the following:

Robert Abrams, M.D., Director, Clinical Research Center, Downstate Medical Center, Brooklyn, New York.

Allan C. Anderson, Executive Director, Strong Memorial Hospital, Rochester, New York.

Virginia Barham, Ph.D., Nursing Education Consultant, State Board of Nurse Registration, San Francisco, California.

Edward G. Benz, The American Society for Hospital Nursing Service Administrators, AHA, and Director of Nursing, Wilmington Medical Center, Wilmington, Delaware.

Louise Carroll, Governing Council of the Association of Hospital Schools, AHA, and Director of Nursing, Community Hospital of Springfield and Clark Counties, Springfield, Ohio.

Margaret Carroll, Deputy Executive Director, ANA, New York, New York.

Earle M. Chapman, M.D., AMA Council of Medical Education, and practitioner of Internal Medicine, Boston, Massachusetts.

Evelyn Cohelan, Ed.D., Third Vice President, ANA, and Director, Graduate Program in Psychiatric Nursing, University of Maryland, Baltimore, Maryland.

Donald Cordes, Chairman, National Assembly of Hospital Schools of Nursing, AHA, and Administrator, Iowa Methodist Hospital, Des Moines, Iowa.

John Danielson, Council of Teaching Hospitals, Association of American Medical Colleges, Washington, D.C.

Grace Davidson, The American Society for Hospital Nursing Service Administrators, AHA, and Division of Nursing, New York University Medical Center, New York, New York.

William DeMaria, M.D., Associate Professor of Pediatrics, Duke University, Durham, North Carolina.

Mary A. Dineen, Ed.D., Director, Department of Baccalaureate and Higher Degree Programs, NLN, New York, New York.

Louis Drexler, Administrator, Worcester Hahnemann Hospital, Worcester, Massachusetts.

Veronica M. Driscoll, Chairman, Commission on Economic and General Welfare, ANA, New York, New York.

Carol M. Eady, Third Vice President, NLN, and Director of Nursing Education, Michael Reese Hospital and Medical Center School of Nursing, Chicago, Illinois.

Leon P. Fox, M.D., AMA Committee on Nursing, and practitioner of Obstetrics and Gynecology, San Jose, California.

William S. Hall, M.D., AMA Committee on Nursing, and Commissioner of Mental Health, State of South Carolina, Columbia, South Carolina.

Adele Herwitz, Associate Executive Director, ANA, New York, New York.

Leah Hornig, Director, Department of Public Health Nursing, NLN, New York, New York.

Charles L. Hudson, M.D., Board of Directors, NLN, and Senior Consultant, Division of Medicine, The Cleveland Clinic, Cleveland, Ohio.

Eileen Jacobi, Ed.D., Associate Executive Director, ANA, New York, New York.

Dorothy E. Johnson, Chairman, ANA Congress for Nursing Practice, and Professor of Nursing, U.C.L.A., Los Angeles, California.

Martha Johnson, Secretary, Council on Nursing, AHA, Chicago, Illinois.

Cynthia R. Kinsella, Ed.D., Vice Chairman, Congress on Nursing Practice, ANA, and Director of Nursing, Mt. Sinai Hospital, New York, New York.

Charles L. Leedham, M.D., Chairman, AMA Committee on Nursing, and Director, Bureau of Educational Activities, Pennsylvania Department of Health, Harrisburg, Pennsylvania.

Gwendoline MacDonald, Ed.D., President, NLN, and Director and Professor of Nursing, Michigan State University, East Lansing, Michigan.

Gladys McGregor, Director, Division of Hospital Schools of Nursing, AHA, Chicago, Illinois.

Marion I. Murphy, Ph.D., Vice-Chairman, ANA Commission on Nursing Education, and Dean, School of Nursing, University of Maryland, Baltimore, Maryland.

Charles Paxson, Governing Council, Association of Hospital Schools, AHA, and Administrator and Vice President, Hahnemann Medical College and Hospital, Philadelphia, Pennsylvania.

Hildegard E. Peplau, Ed.D., Executive Director, ANA, New York, New York.

Martha Pitel, Ph.D., Chairman, Department of Nursing, University of Kansas Medical Center, Kansas City, Kansas.

Muriel A. Poulin, Vice-Chairman, ANA Commission on Economic and General Welfare, and Associate Professor, College of Nursing, University of Kentucky, Lexington, Kentucky.

Eva Reese, Vice-Chairman, ANA Committee on Nursing Services, and Executive Director, Visiting Nurse Service, New York, New York.

E. Bryce Robinson, Jr., M.D., AMA Council on Medical Education, and Medical Director, Lloyd Noland Hospital and Clinic, Fairfield, Alabama.

John Sbarbaro, M.D., Medical Coordinator, Neighborhood Health Programs, Department of Health and Hospitals, Denver, Colorado.

Eugene J. Smith, The American Society of Hospital Nursing Service Administrators, AHA, and Director of Nursing, Charlotte Memorial Hospital, Charlotte, North Carolina.

Adele G. Stahl, Vice-Chairman, ANA Council of State Boards of Nursing, and Department of Regulation and Licensing, Division of Nurses, Madison, Wisconsin.

Gloria Swanberg, President, The American Society of Hospital Nursing Service Administrators, AHA, and Director of Nursing Service, Abbott Hospital, Minneapolis, Minnesota.

Kathleen M. Sward, Vice-Chairman, ANA Congress for Nursing Practice, and Nursing Practice Consultant, Harlem Hospital Center Evaluation Unit, New York, New York.

Margaret E. Walsh, General Director, NLN, New York, New York.

Mamie Wang, Outpatient Nursing Department, The New York Hospital-Cornell Medical Center, New York, New York.

William R. Willard, M.D., Chairman, AMA Council on Medical Education, and Vice President, Medical Center, University of Kentucky, Lexington, Kentucky.

In listing their names here, we do not mean to imply that these individuals agreed entirely with our analyses and recommendations. However, their suggestions and comments contributed immensely to the final drafting of our report. We were able to define our terms and develop our proposals more clearly, and in so doing to meet most, if not all, of the criticisms that came out of these small-group meetings. We trust that many of these individuals will recognize our acceptance and use of their advice.

Thus, the final recommendations of our study evolved from two major sources: the data collected through literature searches, surveys, reviews of past studies, and on-site visits; and the numerous discussions with advisory panelists, conference participants, and invited specialists, as well as staff contacts with thousands of individuals across the country.

PROSPECTS FOR CHANGE

Since 1923 there has been a succession of studies, inquiries, and investigations into nursing in the United States. For the most part, these studies have had limited impact on the profession itself and on related institutions and health care groups. This inaction has stemmed in large measure from inertia. In addition, some antagonism toward change has been generated among the groups that make up the health professions. At times, too, the people involved have failed to see a clear need for innovation. Many of the recommendations have been in advance of their day—so far advanced that they seemed unrelated to the then-current problems of the medical world.

It would seem in 1970 that the times and the conditions are significantly different. First, there is general recognition both within and outside the nursing profession that things must change in order to ensure minimal standards for future patient care. While there may not be consensus on the underlying causes, there is little question in anyone's mind that there is a critical scarcity of nurses having direct contact with patients.

Second, the growing public concern over the costs and conditions of patient service requires that health care professionals place their overriding emphasis on the solutions to nursing's problems before they consider the requirements of individual institutions or specialties. While there are certain differences in state and local concerns, the problems of nursing care are a national phenomenon that requires national attention. The American public, through its increasing awareness of the size of the problem, has been drawn into the process of decision-making and implementation.

Third, this combination of recognized need and increasing public involvement has already begun to have an effect on some of the hardened partisan policies that were adopted in the past. During the 1960's, for example, the American Nurses' Association, the National League for Nursing, the American Medical Association, and the American Hospital Association, along with constituent bodies, engaged in internecine warfare over policy positions in nursing and the proposed solutions to its problems. These groups are now aware that they must resolve their differences in behalf of optimum patient care or they may well lose the opportunity forever as the power of solution is taken out of their hands by the public and its representatives. Fortunately for all concerned, the professions are well aware of the proposed alternatives and have displayed a healthy willingness to compromise.

In the final analysis, change will be accomplished because change is required if we are going to have sufficient numbers of nurses capable of performing their special functions in the care and treatment of patients. Similarly, to ensure that nurses practice to their highest capacity will require change in traditional roles and functions. At present, the braking power of inertia is dead within the health care system. The only question that remains is the manner and direction for change, not whether it should or should not take place. There is also the fact that, in accordance with the Surgeon General's proposal, we now have available an independent analysis of the nursing profession, apart from the parochialism of a single viewpoint. An additional resource is the commitment of this commission, its study staff, and its advisors to see that change does come, and to invest the required effort and time to continue the follow-up activities that are necessary to mount a program of change. The need is here; the recommendations of this report constitute one reasonable path to the goals we seek. Now it is up to all of us to initiate these changes, or, from growing wisdom, to discover and implement better suggestions. The alternative of inaction on nursing's problems could be highly detrimental to our entire system of health care delivery.

SUMMARY

We have described the history and organization of the commission and its study staff. Further, we have identified four key problems in nursing: the continuing disparity between the supply of and demand for nurses; the problems involved in nursing education; the changing roles and functions in nursing practice; and the inherent weaknesses of nursing as a lifetime professional career. Each of these problems has been analyzed during the course of our study.

However fascinating or disturbing the problems of nursing, they must be viewed as an integral part of the entire health care system in the United States. Furthermore, that system has been under stress for the past decade. Since the Second World War, in fact, we have seen dramatic changes in our society, triggered by a population explosion and increased expectation of freely available health care for all citizens. Corresponding changes in population density have taxed the capability of the health system to respond.

Advances in medical science have been remarkable, but even here we find paradox. Increased life expectancy, for example, requires a broad new system of care and institutional living that we have not needed before. Our very success in medical science creates new demands and new problems.

The changed economy of our society, embodied in a situation of full employment, has increased the effective demand for health services. A growing proportion of our gross national product goes into health care. Expanded use of insurance plans for treatment and care has sharply increased our need to provide care for millions of our citizens.

Not one of these trends is reversible. To the contrary, there is every sign that the demands on our health care system will accelerate and widen.

Inevitably, these developments will place a great burden on nursing and the other health professions. At the same time, these trends represent our best guarantee that fundamental changes can take place in nursing education and service to enable nursing to enlarge its contribution—and perhaps ensure that our system for health care will remain viable and responsive to the demands placed upon it.

FOOTNOTES

1. *Toward Quality in Nursing.* Report of the Surgeon General's Consultant Group on Nursing. Washington, D.C.: U.S. Department of Health, Education, and Welfare, Public Health Service, PHS Publication No. 992. 1963. p. 55.
2. *Report of the National Advisory Commission on Health Manpower, Vol. 1.* Washington, D.C.: U.S. Government Printing Office. 1966. p. 2.
3. *Nurse Training Act of 1964, Program Review Report.* Washington, D.C.: U.S. Department of Health, Education, and Welfare, Public Health Service. PHS Publication No. 1740. 1967. p. 9.
4. "The Plight of the U.S. Patient." *Time.* February 21, 1968. p. 54.

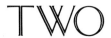

TWO

NURSING IN THE AMERICAN HEALTH SCENE

Since 1798, nurses have helped to provide direct, personal care to the ill and disabled of this country. During these years, the American public has developed a genuine affection and respect for "the lady in white" who has proffered both comfort and care. To the patient, to his family, to the public at large, nursing is a valued occupation—one that many regard as a prime career for the dedicated young woman.

Yet today, that same public senses that nursing is a troubled profession. We hear of nurse shortages, but most of us know inactive nurses who do not care to go back to their occupation. Worse yet, former patients recount unfavorable experiences with the quality and extent of nursing care. As population increases and health care demands expand, the problems become even more pronounced. Duff and Hollingshead recapitulate common experience when they say, "The central purpose of the hospital, i.e., the care of patients, especially the personal aspects of that care, was not controlled directly or effectively by the hospital or anyone."[1] To the man in the street, the nurse is one person who should be able to ensure that individual care *is* provided—ably and personally. When he fails to receive it, he is apt to place the blame on nursing.

While the general public may not be aware of the full impact of the problems facing the profession, there are segments of the population that have had forceful confrontation with these issues. The sight of nurses on picket lines, the spectacle of public controversy over rival professional positions, and the growing militancy of certain nursing spokesmen point up the need for independent assessment of a complex situation.

The place to begin our focus on current problems, it seems to us, is with an examination of nursing's history, its problems and progress, and its aspirations and disappointments.

NURSING AND THE NATION'S HEALTH

Beginning with the development of the first lectures on sick care for attendants at the New York Hospital in 1798, the public has recognized the need for more knowledgeable patient care in the United States. It is noteworthy, however, that 75 years passed before the first training schools for nursing were established. In the interim, individuals and institutions conducted short courses and lecture series to provide nurses for the nation's hospitals. Undoubtedly, the catastrophic impact of the Civil War, coupled with the English experience in the Crimea, helped to secure support for the establishment of the Bellevue Hospital School in 1873.

Today, nurses constitute the largest single group of health professionals involved in patient care. In 1968, for example, there were 659,000 employed registered nurses in the United States. In addition, there were 320,000 practical nurses and 800,000 nurse aides, orderlies, and attendants.[2] In comparison, in 1968 there were 294,100 medical doctors and 11,400 osteopathic physicians.[3]

Of the registered nurses at work in the health fields in 1967, approximately 63 percent were employed in hospitals, 19 percent in private duty or office work, 6 percent in public health, 5 percent in nursing homes, 4 percent in nursing education, and 3 percent in occupational health.[4] Over the past several years, there has been a steady increase in the number of nurses in relation to population; in 1954, for example, there were 251 nurses per 100,000; in 1968, the figure stood at 331 nurses per 100,000.[5]

As both the actual and relative numbers of nurses have grown, there has been a corresponding increase in responsibility and level of practice. Until 1870, the duties of the nurse included care of the patient, sweeping of fireplaces, washing of stairs and dishes, and laundering of bandages so they could be used again.[6] Today, however, we find that the nurse is functioning as the primary health practitioner in an increasing number of instances. At the University of Kansas, for example, nurses perform almost interchangeably with physicians in caring for ambulatory patients;[7] in Denver, nurses with specialized training provide a wide range of primary health service for pediatric patients.[8]

This great range of tasks—from cleaning and housekeeping to diagnosis and treatment—represents both the content and the confusion of nursing today. Nurses themselves perceive that they are often at the center of disparate and competing forces. Undeniably, nursing is the practice of a body of knowledge and skills, designed to be restorative and comforting, to prevent or control disease and disability, and to provide health guidance in concert with other health workers and the physician. At the same time, it is also the performance of diverse and ill-defined functions that "have always been done" or that help to keep the institution "running smoothly."

By their very numbers and deep involvement in the health care system, nurses play an essential part in direct patient care. But what about their performance? In the hospital studied by Duff and Hollingshead, "*. . . nursing care was erratic and usually inadequate.* It is likely to remain so unless sweeping changes are brought about."[9] This is not an isolated observation. The Governor's Committee on Nursing in Virginia examined nursing service throughout the commonwealth and observed, "In summary, responses represented problems that have been present in the hospitals for a number of years and still continue to be present."[10] In a carefully developed analysis of the social and occupational forces that impinge on nursing, Lambertsen found persistent problems in nursing which " . . . have deep roots in the past and are perpetuated through the value placed on tradition."[11]

If there is a deep concern for change in the system of health care in the United States, then nursing is not exempt from the challenge. This need for adjustment has been powerfully stated by Christman:

> "In affluent societies, health and education become prime targets for social concern. When a rapid expansion of knowledge and technology is combined with a state of great affluency, social unrest, mass communication, and a knowledgeable public, a dynamic condition that will markedly change health care practice in the future, is created. A generation ago, nurses could cope very casually with change and the use of new knowledge. . . . No longer will static, settled patterns of nursing practice exist. Instead, the only constant demand will be one of newness."[12]

Other observers have also commented on the need to change the function of nursing and its role in caring for the nation's health. As Dolan points out, "Many nurses today have the necessary knowledge and abilities to expand their roles in the diagnostic, preventive, and therapeutic areas of patient and family care. Many more could be prepared in reasonably short and intensive training programs to fill these roles."[13]

If there are persons in the United States who are not receiving adequate health care, or indeed who receive none at all, can we afford to utilize our largest group of health professionals at anything less than their highest capacity? Perhaps by looking at the historical development of nursing in this country we can understand why we stand where we do today. By studying the patterns of the past, we may be able to answer for ourselves the rhetorical question posed by Duff and Hollingshead: "Shall we complacently continue to 'walk backward into the future,' congratulating ourselves on how much better medical care is today than it was in the early part of this century, or will our challenge be met?"[14]

HISTORICAL DEVELOPMENT OF PROFESSIONAL NURSING[15]

The beginnings of the profession can be traced to the foundation of the Nightingale School of Nursing in London in 1860. Eight years later, the American Medical Association prompted a committee investigation of hospital facilities in the United States. The ensuing report recommended that nursing care be provided by trained attendants and further that district schools be established specifically to provide this training. As early as 1857, the New York Infirmary had offered a free four-month course in nursing, and similar programs soon followed in Philadelphia and Boston. It was in 1872 that the first class of "trained nurses" graduated from the school of the New England Hospital for Women and Children. In the next year, three training schools based on the English model were established at Bellevue, New Haven, and Massachusetts General.

These early institutions prepared only women to become nurses. In part, this practice stemmed from outright medical opposition to the acceptance of women as medical students or doctors (it was not until 1876 that a woman was allowed to join the American Medical Association). A related reason, however, was the early identification of nursing with the suffragette movement. Elizabeth Blackwell, the first woman to graduate from medical school in the United States, was the founder of the New York Infirmary and a confidante of Lucy Stone and Susan B. Anthony, perhaps the most prominent leaders in the struggle for women's rights. Nursing early became one of the "respectable occupations" for girls, and one of the few alternatives that lay open to those who wanted a career.

The fundamental tie between the hospital and the school of nursing proved to be a strong influence on the way that students were trained. A leading figure in the development of nursing schools wrote, "The superintendent of a training-school is under a threefold obligation: first, to the hospital where she works; secondly, to the patients who are entrusted to her care; and thirdly, to the women for whose education as nurses she is responsible."[16] The priority of concerns speaks for itself.

In the nineteenth century, the professional avenues open to women were extremely limited. In fact, the first association organized and controlled by women was the American Society of Superintendents of Training Schools for Nurses of the United States and Canada, founded in 1894. Through a series of changes and mergers, this became, in 1952, the National League for Nursing, an organization that continues today. The Nurses Associated Alumnae of the United States and Canada (note the Latin plural feminine ending) was organized in 1897 and became, in 1912, the American Nurses' Association. Today this body is the largest professional women's organization in the world, though its membership includes male nurses as well.

The response to the new nursing programs was quite beyond the dreams of the innovators. While doctors might resent a woman as a colleague, they valued her as an aide. Moreover, the location of a school of nursing in conjunction with a hospital was seen as a worthwhile investment, for it provided both a source of ready student labor and a vocational orientation to continued work in the same hospital. Whatever the motives of their founders, the growth of these schools was phenomenal. In 1900 there were 432 schools of nursing; by 1910, the figure stood at 1,105; in 1920, the total was 1,755; and by 1931, the number of schools rose to an all-time high of 1,844. The length of their courses ranged from six weeks to three years, and it is probably well within the mark to say that the quality of instruction was at least as different as its duration.

So great were the disparities among these institutions that by 1900 there were efforts underway to fix professional standards for nursing education. In 1903, in fact, North Carolina enacted the first nurse registration law that set minimum standards of competence. Gradually other states followed suit, but there continued to be remarkable differences in regulations. Even today, eight states still allow voluntary licensure, which enables unlicensed persons to practice, but does forbid them from using the title of nurse.

Related to the campaign for registration and licensure, there was an active attempt by nurses to improve the quality of the faculty, and thereby the instruction, in the preparatory schools. Beginning in 1899, Teachers College of Columbia University provided a series of courses for graduate nurses in such fields as psychology, educational methods, and training school management. In 1907 a Division of Hospital Economics was added, the course was lengthened to two years, and graduates received a bachelor of science degree.

In this same period, the head of the Johns Hopkins Training School recommended to the board of trustees that "careful attention . . . be given to the more purely intellectual part of the nurse's training to the end that nursing may be elevated to a profession and raised as far as possible above the status of a mere trade."[17] It was not suggested, however, that nurses enroll in the university courses or receive a university degree. Thus, by the early 1900's there was a fundamental split in the ranks of nursing over the proper location of nursing education. Some who wanted to increase professionalism sought inclusion in institutions of higher education; others set out to improve the quality of instruction within the environment of the hospital system.

It is seldom recognized that the developments in nursing education closely parallel those in the medical schools. In 1905, for example, only five of 160 medical schools required graduation from college. Before that time, only a few schools required a high school diploma, and many courses of instruction lasted just two years. Medicine did not incorporate actual hospital experience into its curriculum until well into the twentieth century, sometime after the clinical demonstration of nursing procedures was an established part of nurse training. It is fair to say that in 1900 there was less difference between the education of the doctor and the nurse than many realize—or some like to accept.

In the midst of struggles to consolidate the position and improve the education of nurses, there were also strenuous efforts to extend their work outside the general hospital. In 1902 the first school nurses were employed in New York City; in 1909 the Metropolitan Life Insurance Company inaugurated the visiting nurse service. Public health had become a field of such interest and activity for nurses that a national organization was established in 1912. In the main, however, just as today, most nurses were employed by hospitals or served as private duty nurses in hospitals and homes.

An important step in nursing education came in 1909 when the University of Minnesota established the first collegiate school of nursing in the United States. The program required three years, and the graduates received a diploma—not a degree. This pattern was followed by a number of other colleges and universities. In 1916, Teachers College and the School of Nursing at the Presbyterian Hospital in New York City established a five-year program leading to the baccalaureate degree in nursing. That same year, the University of Cincinnati founded a similar five-year program. In 1923, the first independent professional school of nursing was established at Yale University to accept arts and science graduates and develop them as nurses. Although the growth of collegiate programs in nursing has seemed slow and faltering at times, there were more than 170 institutions accredited by the National League for Nursing in 1969 for baccalaureate and/or masters degree programs in nursing.

From the high point of 1,844 preparatory programs in nursing in 1931, there was a steady decline through the depression years and even following the Second World War to a low of 1,114 in 1960. Most of the closings came as a result of economic exigency, and the effect was most dramatic on the hospital schools.

After 1960, the number of nurse preparatory programs began to climb again. There were 1,145 in 1964, 1,219 in 1966, and 1,269 in 1967. This growth can be attributed to an increase in the number of collegiate programs and to a large expansion in associate degree, or junior college, programs. In this latter category there were fewer than 50 in 1958; more than 300 existed by 1968. Obviously, their growth·is the primary reason for the overall increase in the number of available nursing courses. While most of the junior college programs stem from the last decade, there were some 12 nursing school-junior college affiliations in 1931; during the same year only 55 nursing school-college affiliations were in operation.

For reasons we will discuss later, the decline in the number of hospital diploma schools has continued while the collegiate programs have expanded. In 1960, for example, there were more than 900 hospital schools; in 1967, 767 remained—a drop of approximately 16 percent.

With the increase in collegiate nursing programs, in both the number and variety of institutions, there has been growing concern with the content and structure of the curriculum. While licensure might control the most obvious failings, it remained an essentially negative screen, and the leaders in nursing sought to develop a more positive thrust. In 1917, a *Standard Curriculum for Schools of Nursing*[18] was distributed by the National League for Nursing Education. Ten years later the League's *A Curriculum for Schools of Nursing*[19] appeared; this document, in turn, was revised and reissued in 1937. These guides were regarded as statements of minimum standards, and were widely used as a basis for assessing nursing courses throughout the world.

Despite the obvious strides that nurses made in establishing themselves as members of a profession, it is ironic that two world wars may have played a more significant role than any other factor in helping nurses to reach their goal. The accomplishments of nurses in the First World War led to their receiving "relative" rank in the Army; this did not deter the United States Civil Service Commission from classifying nurses as subprofessionals in 1923. The proportionally greater involvement of nurses in all the armed forces in the Second World War led to their receiving permanent commissions, and, in 1947, to their classification as professionals by the Civil Service Commission. National need and the effective response of nursing had led to the recognition that nursing leadership alone could not attain.

Throughout this period, starting with the Goldmark report of 1923,[20] a number of nursing studies appeared, including the Brown report of 1948,[21] the Ginzberg report of 1949,[22] the Montag study of 1951,[23] and the Bridgman study of 1953.[24] These will be treated at length in subsequent sections of this report, but the number and frequency of these projects attest to the persistence of problems in the nursing profession.

CURRENT PROBLEMS AND TRENDS IN NURSING[25]

Nursing stands at a critical point in American history. Because it is an integral part of the entire health industry, nursing is affected by the major movements within our society, in general, and within the health system, in particular. Any consideration of the problems and trends of nursing apart from these powerful currents is unrealistic. These forces have been summarized by Anderson[26] as follows:

a. The population will continue to grow in the foreseeable future. This will cause both an absolute and a relative increase in those portions of the population that are high users of health service.

b. The economy will continue to expand resulting in an increased gross national product and increased discretionary income in both the public and private sectors. Money will be less of a concern though priorities of expenditure will continue to be matters for argument.

c. Medical technology will increase in size, complexity, and effectiveness in saving and prolonging life. Many of the people whose lives are extended or saved, however, will require never-ending, closely supervised medical care.

d. There will also be an increase in the number of people requiring long-term and basic, custodial care.

e. The unit cost of personnel will increase in order to compete with the labor market, and this will intensify the desire for substitutions for registered nurses and will give the registered nurse an increasingly higher status.

f. Associated with this last trend will be an increasing differentiation among registered nurses in clinical specialties.

g. Women of high school age aspiring for professional status will do so through the avenue of the college or university rather than through institutions associated with vocational training.

h. The qualifications for professional attainment will continue to emphasize technical proficiency based on physical and natural sciences rather than nurturance based on behavioral science, feeling, and compassion. This will be one of the problems the nursing profession must watch diligently as it aspires toward higher professional status.

i. The quality and skill of the managers of the health services system will continue to improve. This will result in greater effectiveness, but not necessarily less cost.

The problems that nursing faces today must also be considered in terms of its efforts to stand as a professional body, a mature contributor to the nation's health needs. If we examine nursing in the light of the common characteristics of professional groups, we can better understand the reasons for much of the disagreement that currently exists. These common characteristics include level of commitment, disciplined educational process, unique body of knowledge and skill, active and cohesive professional organization, and discretionary authority and judgment.

Level of Commitment

A profession is commonly distinguished by the fact that its members engage in active pursuit of their occupation during most of their lives. By such a standard, nursing is certainly placed in an ambivalent position. Setting aside the fact that approximately one-third of those students in preparatory nursing programs drop out before completion of their course, it has been shown that nurses leave their profession at a much higher rate than physicians, engineers, lawyers, or teachers.

In 1966, for example, there were 909,131 nurses in the United States. Of these, 65.3 percent were employed in nursing; 31.4 percent were not employed in nursing; and 3.3 per cent constituted an unreported category. Of those who were employed in nursing, approximately 445,300 were working full-time and 148,000 were working part-time. In effect, the number of registered nurses employed full-time in their profession represented only 49 percent of the total.[27] In contrast, it is reported that 88 percent of women M.D.'s are practicing medicine, the majority of them full-time.[28]

Despite the fairly low percentage of registered nurses who are employed full-time at any given period, there is evidence that many nurses do work for a substantial number of years, and that the supplemental activity of the part-time nurse contributes a significant number of man-years. The federal Bureau of Health Manpower has estimated that the average working life of a nurse is between 20 and 21 years.[29] This figure is at one and the same time larger than might be guessed from some of the statements appearing in the press about nurse manpower, and small by comparison to the years that might be expected from looking at other professions. For example, a nurse graduating at age 21 might anticipate some 44 years of professional work before customary retirement at age 65. The highest estimate of professional working life, 21 years, would constitute 48 percent of the "total available time."

Of course, when we examine a statement such as "nurses will remain active professionals throughout life," we must conclude that the basic premise is untrue, and is likely to remain untrue. After all, nursing is a woman's occupation. Approximately 99 percent of the registered nurses in active practice are women. As a result, nurses in particular are subject to all the interruptions that might be expected in their professional employment as a result of child-bearing, family rearing, and other marital responsibilities. Of the registered nurses under age 30, for example, 95 percent of those who are unmarried are professionally employed. Only 64 percent of the married nurses in the same age group are in practice.

Trends for the future are unclear. There is a steady increase in the number and percentage of part-time nurses returning to professional work. This group represented 18 percent of the employed nurses in 1960; 23 percent in 1964; and,

in 1969, 25 percent of the working nurses. It is this return of the part-time, previously inactive nurse that is largely credited with the increased supply of nurses
over the past few years.[30] This pattern may well be crucial for the future. The
United States leads all western nations both in an increasing marriage rate and in
a lowered age at which marriage takes place.[31] As Glaser points out, "Surveys
of undergraduate nursing students show that all desire and expect marriage during
and soon after nursing school, virtually all expect to give marriage and mother-
hood priority over nursing work . . . ."[32]

Thus, we may expect that American nurses will continue in a cycle of full-
time work immediately after graduation, resignation during pregnancy and child-
rearing, then a return to part-time work for varying, but perhaps lengthy, periods
of time. This may well satisfy certain manpower needs, but does it allow for professionalism? Glaser, for one, feels that "the leaders of nursing have wanted
their followers to become successful professionals, but instead American nurses
seem to have become successful and satisfied American women."[33]

Many of the dire predictions of nurse shortages, and many of the actual cases
of closing of wards due to a lack of nursing personnel, can be traced to the large
percentage of inactive nurses. In Chapter Three we shall look at the projections
for manpower requirements, but we should point out that nursing may expect more
difficulties in the future than it has experienced in the past because of its nearly
complete reliance on women to populate the profession.

As Anderson emphasizes, ". . . the health services system . . . is no longer in
a favored position to attract women into the nursing services as one of only two or
three alternatives . . . ."[34] An increasing number of occupational and career alternatives plus a rise in standard and competitive wages has enlarged the horizons
of women seeking employment. If there truly was a time when nursing and school
teaching represented the major career choices for women, then we must conclude
that we have another era entirely.

Anderson goes on to cite three historic conditions that tend to inhibit the
choice of nursing as a professional career: the relatively poor salary in the health
services system; the shift from "acute and dramatic disease episodes" toward the
care of patients suffering long-term, intractable illness with the resultant increase
in tedium; and a growing disdain in our society for any jobs of a servant nature.[35]

In terms of the present idiom, nursing just may not appeal to as many girls
as it once did, and its attractiveness as a professional career may suffer greatly,
in contrast to its utility as a part-time vocation for the later years of a woman's
life. One piece of evidence that substantiates this belief is the slight but steady
decrease in the percentage of high school graduates who choose nursing as a
career. In 1957, nursing was the career choice of 6 percent of the girl graduates;
by 1967, it had declined to only 4.5 percent. This trend is generally obscured by

population growth and the increased size of the graduating classes that result in larger numbers of entering students despite the relative loss of popularity of nursing as a career.[36]

At this time, we are unable to specify to what extent the very functions of nursing adversely affect the commitment to a professional career. Many observers agree, however, that this is an important factor. Davis, Olesen, and Whittaker state, ". . . one of the more persistent themes to emerge from our field work is that of the progressive disenchantment of students with hospital nursing . . . ."[37] This would seem to be the thrust of the Willard report[38] when it characterized nursing as "a fragmented, task oriented service."

One final aspect of the woman-nurse factor in relation to professional commitment may be seen in the mobility and geographic distribution of active registered nurses. In common with the population as a whole, nurses have tended to move into urban and suburban areas and away from rural parts of the country. This trend has seriously affected the relative availability of nurses, with the New England region having 509 nurses to each 100,000 population, and the East South Central region having only 176 nurses per 100,000.[39] Moreover, most hospitals commonly experience high rates of turnover each year as nurses enter and leave the labor force or simply move to other institutions. Frequently, turnover ratio runs as high as 50 to 75 percent, with some hospitals facing a change in nursing personnel of more than 100 percent during a 12-month period. To some extent, both availability and turnover result as the married nurse follows the career choice and opportunities of her husband. Given the fact that young nursing students place family above profession, it is not at all surprising that decisions on where to practice are determined, for the most part, by family priorities.

In short, while there are large numbers of highly committed nurses within the profession, there are still reasons for skepticism over the depth of this commitment throughout the rank and file. Glaser observes that "the leaders of the professional movement in American nursing were always ahead of most nurses, but . . . social change may have taken the bulk of the occupation in another direction."[40] By this he means that the majority of nurses have chosen to play the role of wife and mother first and to find in these functions the rewards that others find in professional pursuits. The nursing leadership must address this problem squarely; the future of the profession depends on the continued and deepened commitment of an ever-increasing number of nurses.

Long and Disciplined Educational Process

The second characteristic common to the professions is that of education — a lengthy and rigorous process that incorporates both theoretical and applied content. Throughout the history of American nursing, individuals have striven to change and improve the content, and the processes, of nursing education. Only the uninitiated observer, however, could feel that the results have been satisfactory and the major problems solved.

Before the establishment of the New Training Schools in 1873, nursing had been largely a vocational skill, acquired through short training periods, a few lectures, and a great deal of on-the-job experience, gathered in an 80- to 90-hour week. While Bellevue and its sister establishments offered an improvement over what had existed, the proliferation of hospital schools was accompanied by great disparities in training and education. It was a reaction to this state of affairs that prompted the creation of the *Standard Curriculum for Schools of Nursing* in 1917 in an effort to set forth the acceptable standards for nursing education.

After some months, leaders in the profession began to wonder whether the standard curriculum was being applied. Their concern led to a conference on the problems and issues, and, in 1920, to the formation of a Committee for the Study of Nursing Education. The committee document, known as the Goldmark report, was published in 1923 and was quite critical of the state of nursing education. The report stressed, in particular, the problematic, dual role of the hospital nursing schools. The hospital schools had two responsibilities: to educate nurses and to provide nursing service to patients. When these two aims were in conflict, the requirements for service predominated and the needs of education yielded.[41]

The report went on to say that many of the schools, approximately 40 percent, were too small to offer adequate experience, and that most schools demonstrated shortcomings in the quality of instruction and the articulation between classroom and nursing assignments.[42]

Twenty-five years later, working independently, Esther Lucile Brown still found a wide range of quality and content among the hospital schools of nursing.[43] Still later, in 1953, Bridgman found widespread evidence of poor teaching, repetitive practice of techniques, and insufficient emphasis on the educational purposes of the school.[44] Writing in 1968, Anderson can look back on this succession of investigations and say, "The great bulk of the nurses are still being trained in diploma schools associated with hospitals and largely on an apprenticeship basis with unsystematic exposures to theoretical and tested knowledge."[45]

We must point out, however, that Goldmark, Brown, Bridgman, and, perhaps by inference, Anderson made sharp discriminations among several levels of quality within the hospital schools. Brown, in particular, spoke of *"Distinguished Hospital Schools."* Nevertheless, there was consistency among the studies in recommending changes in the educational system, with a specific suggestion that institutions of higher education become more involved in the development of nurses.

As a reaction to these findings, and in an overt effort to increase professionalism and thus improve practice, a growing number of leaders in nursing insisted that nursing education be housed in the junior and senior colleges of the country. A corollary of this proposal, of course, was that the educational process should become "longer and more disciplined" in accordance with the characteristics of a profession. (Even in those cases in which a junior college program might be shorter in total length than a hospital school program, the academic instruction in the collegiate course was intended to be longer, with a corresponding reduction in service and practice time.) As Rogers states it, "Professional education requires rigorous intellectual training. A body of abstract principles, the product of scientific research and logical analysis, is indispensable to its being."[46] She then adds, "Professional education of any quality is an integral part of higher education."[47]

With the establishment of the Division of Hospital Economics at Teachers College in 1907 and the inauguration of the University of Minnesota School of Nursing in 1909, the first steps were underway to develop professional nursing programs within a collegiate setting. It was 1916 before the first degree programs were offered in nursing at Yale and Cincinnati. Since then, the growth and extension of collegiate nursing programs have been far from revolutionary, but there has been a steady increase. In the five-year period from 1962 to 1967, for example, the number of collegiate schools rose from 170 to 214, a gain of 44 and an average increase of almost nine schools a year.[48]

If some nursing leaders thought that nursing education within the college environment would solve the professional problems, they were headed for disappointment. When Bridgman reviewed collegiate education for nursing in 1953, she found a large number of difficulties. She argued that "many colleges and universities have misunderstood the purpose of higher education in nursing . . . . Many educators tend to think of nursing education only as 'training' . . . colleges [are] establishing affiliation with individual hospital schools, without investigation or concern about educational standards."[49] She underscores the point that the entire purpose of collegiate preparation is defeated ". . . unless policies applied to nursing are consistent with general standards of colleges and universities."[50] Obviously, she found severe shortcomings.

Strauss feels that collegiate nursing is still hampered by a number of problems: a variety of educational institutions and degrees; the low academic prestige of nursing within the college or university; a heritage of affiliation with the professional schools of education; and the induced strain between practitioners who came from diploma schools and educators who are intent on eliminating any but collegiate schools of nursing.[51]

Within the collegiate schools, there is no common agreement on what constitutes the content of the "long and disciplined educational process." Even as a few schools are beginning major curricular overhauling, some critics are suggesting that the collegiate schools are preparing "well-rounded nurse generalists" when they should be producing "highly skilled specialists."[52] Similarly, there are criticisms of the separation of collegiate nursing education from nursing practice and direct patient care—the feeling that the collegiate educators have overplayed their hands in divorcing nursing education from the hospital or from other care facilities.[53]

Perhaps the most ubiquitous criticism of the present state of nursing education as a professional discipline is the lack of research in that discipline and in the institutional system for providing it. There is general acceptance of the fact that research within nursing has been too little and too weak, and that no disciplined educational process can emerge until more knowledge is acquired. Strauss argues forcefully that "research should be an institutionalized aspect of nursing."[54] He adds that this can be done in a meaningful way only when (a) nursing education and nursing service can be brought closely together within the university teaching hospitals; and (b) clinical innovation in nursing is made a deliberately guided process, associated especially with higher education in nursing.

In short, then, there are difficulties in nursing education that stem from the location, the content, and the development of content. Furthermore, these problems stack up against nursing in its effort to satisfy the professional characteristic of a "long and disciplined educational process." Clearly, the trend is toward a greater utilization of institutions of higher education; the trend is less clear when we examine the need for a rapprochement between education and service that will strengthen meaningful research into the form and content of nursing education.

Unique Body of Knowledge and Skill

One of the most persistent problems faced by nursing is that of defining what nursing is, and what is distinctive about it. This, of course, stems from the close historical relationship between medicine and nursing, both of them involved in the clinical care of a patient. The dilemma has been heightened by the frequent attempts to define nursing in terms of procedures or techniques that emphasize skill at the expense of knowledge or understanding. For example, *An Activity Analysis of Nursing,* published in 1932, listed 659 activities in which nurses were engaged.[55]

Nursing care is related to medical care, and the demarcation between the two professions might be likened to a Venn diagram in which there are both intersections and mutual subsets: a patient might be receiving care during a specified period of time from a physician, a nurse, a therapist, and a fellow family member. For instance, there will be times when the physician or the nurse will perform some acts in the absence of the therapist that the former would not do if he were present. Similarly, there are some acts that would be performed only by one specialist, and

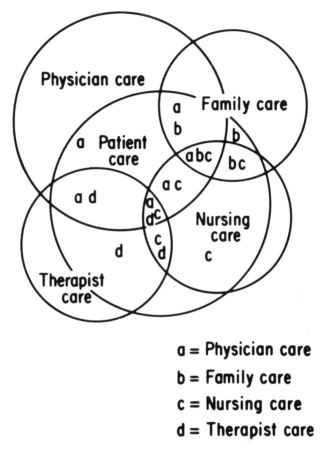

a = Physician care

b = Family care

c = Nursing care

d = Therapist care

Figure 1. Relationship between nursing care and medical care.

these will not be carried out in his absence. Each specialty has a certain body of knowledge and skill that is unique and will not be utilized in the absence of that practitioner. The amount of overlap varies greatly, conditioned as it is by experience, skill, the nature of the patient's problem, and the existing relationships among the principals involved.

As Glaser points out, "It has been easy to define the areas of special nursing competence." He goes on to say, "But every profession depends on the knowledge accumulated through research and writing, and in this respect, the basis of American professional nursing has been stunted." He concludes these remarks with the observation that "because so many nurses are preoccupied with family and nursing service, and because so few American women have yet developed scientific writing skills the growth of nursing science may remain retarded for some time."[56]

In addition to the reiterated need for research to give depth and quality to the body of nursing knowledge, there are particular aspects of the field that have limited its generation of information about itself. Strauss suggests that nursing has too frequently followed ". . . the hierarchical lines of hospitals or agencies and the clinical specializations of medicine."[57] In developing an approach to research and practice, nursing should not be slavish to the current models, either for institutions or for personnel. Speaking to this very point, Anderson says, "The challenge to collegiate nursing is then immense. If the medical specialist becomes the model, the behavioral aspects of patient care will languish and be preempted by lesser trained nurse types, de facto. If the patient-as-a-person orientation can be the model, then, it would seem, professional nursing has a viable role model to develop in its educational program."[58]

It is this search for its unique but complementary role that nursing must now undertake. To develop a truly professional body of knowledge and skill, better research must take place within better drawn limits so that results will be reliable, valid, and applicable to the broad spectrum of nursing problems.

Furthermore, it is essential that the analysis of nursing knowledge and skills be done in the context of increased dialogue between nursing service and education. As Davis, Olesen, and Whittaker emphasize in arguing for a better interface between these two areas, ". . . the nursing profession is admirably suited to combine the complex technical expertise which will be needed with a decent, humanistic regard for patients as persons. But, for this to come about, nursing's leading educational arm, the collegiate school, will have to meet the challenge of technical specialization-in-depth in a more concerted fashion than it has thus far."[59]

Finally, the profession must recognize that nurses teach and administer, as well as provide bedside care. Strauss argues that these quite different functional groupings ". . . have been characteristically blurred, but now are becoming increasingly distinct."[60] We would add only that not all teaching or administration involves dimensions that are unique to nursing. By this we suggest that nursing must determine what aspects of administration are really a valid concern of nursing, and what aspects are more properly assigned to research specialists in business administration, public administration, or other academic disciplines. Development of a "unique body of skills and knowledge" implies thoughtful exclusion as well as intelligent inclusion.

Discretionary Authority and Judgment

The fourth characteristic of a profession is that the practitioners possess and exercise authority and judgment.

Nursing has traditionally been "embedded within a hierarchy of authority" in which its autonomy has been largely circumscribed.[61] Most of the medical and nurse practice acts now written place a sharp limitation on the authority and judgmental exercise of the nurse. In day-to-day situations, however, Hughes has recorded that doctors frequently fail to fully exercise their authority and judgment and that the nurse has to exercise more than is legally reserved to her.[62]

As clinical specialization increases in nursing, there will be a host of questions raised about authority and judgment. The resolution will have profound effects on the profession of nursing—and of medicine.[63] Law and tradition hold that nurses do not make diagnoses. Aside from what a nurse must and will do when no doctor is available for a patient in critical need, there is evidence in the work of a cardiopulmonary specialist or in the decision-making of a pediatric nurse clinician that diagnoses are being made, on some plane and to some degree, and that these practices cannot be ignored.

To consider nursing as a profession in terms of "discretionary authority and judgment," we must discriminate between what law and tradition say; what doctors and nurses do; and, ultimately, what the developing health system will require. In general, legislation follows practice, and practice can only follow education and training. When nursing meets the requirements for professional recognition on the counts of educational process and a unique body of knowledge, then it can be assumed that practice must and will follow.

It is essential, however, that action—not inertia—hold sway and that nurses seek the legal authority commensurate with their responsibility and performance in the developing health system. In this regard, nursing must create awareness of the need for change among other professions, state legislatures, and the public.

Active and Cohesive Professional Organization

The final characteristic of a profession is the presence of a professional association that is cohesive, self-governing, and a source of professional self-discipline, standards, and ethics.

It would seem that the American Nurses' Association should meet these criteria, within such limitations as the uniqueness of nursing and its relationship to other professions, particularly medicine. Here again, we find nursing struggling toward, but not yet attaining, a completely successful professional association that is characteristic of other disciplines.

True, the ANA is the primary national organization for professional nurses, and is strongly engaged through its committees, commissions, and central staff in efforts related to education, practice, and nursing careers. However, in 1967 there were only 204,704 registered nurses who held membership in the association. This represents less than 25 percent of the registered nurses in the United States. On the plus side, the proportion of active nurses who held ANA membership may be considerably higher, and the size of the organization is growing dramatically, as shown by an 18 percent increase in membership in 1967. Furthermore, this trend may continue if we can judge by the increased membership in the National Student Nurses' Association. This organization, which might indicate the depth of future professional involvement, now lists a membership of more than 72,000 from a total enrollment of 142,000 nursing students in the United States—approximately 51 percent participation. Both in size and in percentage of members, the NSNA has been on the rise.[64]

In a recent informal survey of nurses conducted by members of the Texas Nursing Students' Association, questions were asked about the lack of participation in the ANA. The responses indicated that "the major reason was the . . . 'poor image' of the organization." Nurses did not feel, for example, that the organization benefited the individual; some expressed dismay at the level of dues; and others cited disenchantment with meetings and programs sponsored by the organization or its affiliates.[65]

However valid these feelings are, and however representative they might be, we are concerned that the ANA, as the national organization for professional nurses, seek to represent a far greater proportion of American nurses.

In addition to the weakness in membership, the ANA faces some problems that are different from those encountered by other professional organizations. For example, nursing has relatively open recruitment and enrollment. There are more openings in schools of nursing than there are students seeking to attend. This is in sharp contrast to schools of medicine, for example, where approximately half the fully qualified candidates for admission are turned away for lack of space. This permits medicine, then, to select its students and to appraise professional commitment as an important factor in admissions.

In addition, nursing encompasses large numbers of auxiliaries and paraprofessionals who may or may not share nursing's professional concern but who are ineligible for membership in the ANA. Beginning with the first course in practical nursing in 1890, there has been an unending struggle over the roles, the education, and the control of various aides to nursing. Today, there are more than 320,000 practical nurses; 800,000 aides, attendants, and orderlies; and over 12,000 home health aides. By force of numbers, these groups must be considered *vis à vis* professionalism in nursing. It seems quite obvious that their future is intimately bound with that of nursing, and that recommendations for career ladders and future roles must be developed with consideration for these persons and their contributions to patient care.

Nursing, further, has a unique situation to consider: the existence of another national organization that appears to serve many of the same functions as the American Nurses' Association. The National League for Nursing is an organization that was restructured in 1952 to continue the work of the National League of Nursing Education and incorporate several other bodies that had existed separately. The National League includes both individual and agency members. More importantly, however, its membership includes representatives from nursing, practical nursing, aides and orderlies, allied health professions, and lay bodies.

The NLN, through its committees and constituent bodies, maintains programs in nursing education and nursing service that are related to the goals and programs of the ANA. Additionally, the NLN serves its other members in areas outside the interests or purview of the ANA. The distribution of functions and activities does not fit into a tidy picture.

Accreditation, one of the prime functions of most professional bodies, has resided traditionally with the League rather than the Association. One of the concerns for the future of the profession must be its stance toward the continuing relationship and activities of these two national groups.

Most professional organizations also have a major role in achieving prestige for their members and in determining to some extent the distribution of rewards within the profession. The American Association of University Professors, for example, publishes an annual listing and grading of institutions in terms of their compensation practices for faculty. In recent years, the ANA has become much more militant in matters of salary and benefits, and has used a number of tactics to apply pressure on hospitals and administrators who fail to meet salary demands.[66] In some cases, the points of argument covered nursing service and the conditions of patient care as well as basic money concerns.[67] This forceful approach to pay and working conditions has not always found favor with those inside and outside nursing—some find it closer to the work of a labor union than a professional group—but this tactic has succeeded in improving salary levels, and most likely accounts for some of the increased membership in recent years.

While nursing has become more vigorous in economic matters, the profession as a whole has become more and more a salaried occupation. Within nursing, the largest percentage drop in any employment category has been in the number of private duty nurses, the entrepreneurs who have contracted privately for their services. The percentage of nurses employed by hospitals or by other health facilities has expanded correspondingly. This would suggest that economic concerns will continue to occupy a large portion of the ANA's annual program.

A final consideration in the area of professional organization and development is that nursing must concern itself with the specific need to recruit added numbers of leaders. In his examination of nursing leadership and policy, Glaser suggests that there has been a cleavage between the small leadership group in American nursing and the great body of registered nurses in the country.[68] Looking into another aspect of the same problem, Davis, Olesen, and Whittaker summarize their conclusions in this way:

> "Clearly, these findings, as well as corroborative ones from our extensive field work with students, throw into question the belief and claim that collegiate nursing prepares a broad-based leadership corps, as it were for the profession. Again, if by leadership we mean no more than a generalized capacity to assume the initiative in a variety of group endeavors, however and whenever they occur, then doubtlessly these students are as well endowed on the average as other young women and, quite possibly, more so, given their secure backgrounds, greater education, and successful coping with the traumas associated with nursing the sick. Nevertheless, from a structural standpoint, their life style, work and career perspectives augur poorly for their ever assuming strategic positions of organizational power within nursing, positions from which leadership can be exercised in a concerted and broadly consequential way."[69]

Thus, we come almost full circle. We have pointed out the series of deficiencies that still face nursing; we have recognized that commitment to a profession, enhanced education, further research into its unique core of knowledge, and growth of a professional body all require strong leadership. Now, we must face the fact that nursing sees its own leadership group as small in number and hampered by difficulties in developing its own replacements.

These shortcomings and constraints must influence the recommendations for nursing practice, nursing education, and nursing careers in the years ahead.

SUMMARY

Nursing shares both the problems and the opportunities of the health care system in the United States. The history of nursing in this country is marked by progress against great difficulty, by repeated efforts to professionalize, and by frequent instances in which basic decisions about nursing were made by organizations and events outside the profession—leaving the nurses to adjust to them as well as they could.

As we project into the future, we find that nursing has many miles to go before it can reach full professional status. However, its own needs and the health care requirements of the public demand that we begin now to chart a course that will enable the nurses of this country to make the most effective contribution possible to health. And this, in turn, means that nursing must become a full and vital partner in the decisions that affect its future.

FOOTNOTES

1. Duff, R. S. and Hollingshead, A. B. *Sickness and Society.* New York: Harper & Row. 1968. p. 375.

2. *Health Resources Statistics.* Washington, D.C.: U.S. Department of Health, Education, and Welfare, Public Health Service. PHS Publication No. 1509. 1968. p. 135.

3. *Ibid.,* p. 124. (Note: These figures are derived by subtracting the inactive and status-not-reported doctors from the totals of all physicians. The resultant total of 305,500 compares with the reported total of all active physicians quite closely, the tabular figure being shown as 305,453. It should be recognized that not all the active physicians are involved in patient care; some 20,100 are identified as being engaged in "other professional activity," which includes teaching, administration, and research.)

4. American Nurses' Association. *Facts About Nursing, 1968 Edition.* New York: American Nurses' Association. 1968. p. 12.

5. *Ibid.,* p. 10.

6. Bullough, V. L. and Bullough, B. *The Emergence of Modern Nursing. Second Edition.* New York: The Macmillan Company. 1969. p. 128.

7. Lewis, C. E. "The Dynamics of Nursing in Ambulatory Patient Care." Final Report, U.S. Public Health Service Grant NU-00145, *mimeo.,* undated.

8. Silver, H. K., Ford, L. C., and Day, L. R. "The Pediatric Nurse-Practitioner Program." *Journal of the American Medical Association.* 204:4:298. April 22, 1968.

9. Duff, R. S. and Hollingshead, A. B., *op. cit.,* p. 384.

10. Governor's Committee on Nursing. *Nursing in Virginia.* Richmond, Va.: State Council of Higher Education for Virginia. 1969. p. 22.

11. Lambertsen, E. *Education for Nursing Leadership.* Philadelphia: J. B. Lippincott Company. 1958. p. 7.

12. Christman, L. "What the Future Holds for Nursing." Paper presented at the California Regional Medical Program's National Regional Medical Program Conference for Allied Health Professions, April 23, 1969, Pacific Grove, California, *mimeo.,* p. 3.

13. Dolan, M. B. "More Nurses: Better Nursing." Paper presented at the National League for Nursing Biennial Convention, Detroit, Michigan, May 21, 1969. *mimeo.,* p. 7.

14. Duff, R. S. and Hollingshead, A. B., *op. cit.,* p. 385.

15. Throughout this section of the chapter, we have relied heavily upon Bullough, V. L. and Bullough, B. *The Emergence of Modern Nursing, Second Edition.* New York: The Macmillan Company. 1969.

16. Strauss, A. "The Structure and Ideology of American Nursing: An Interpretation." in Davis, F. (Ed.) *The Nursing Profession.* New York: John Wiley & Sons. 1966. pp. 69–70.

17. *Ibid.,* p. 69.

18. National League of Nursing Education. *Standard Curriculum for Schools of Nursing. A Report Prepared by the Committee on Education.* Baltimore: Waverly Press. 1917.

19. National League of Nursing Education. *A Curriculum for Schools of Nursing. A Report Prepared by the Committee on Education.* New York: National League of Nursing Education. 1927.

20. Goldmark, J. *Nursing and Nursing Education in the United States.* New York: The Macmillan Company. 1923.

21. Brown, E. L. *Nursing for the Future.* New York: Russell Sage Foundation. 1948.

22. The Committee on the Function of Nursing. *A Program for the Nursing Profession.* New

York: The Macmillan Company. 1949. (Note: This is commonly known as the Ginzberg Report because of the leadership supplied by Dr. Eli Ginzberg in the work of the committee.)

23. Montag, M. *Education of Nursing Technicians.* New York: G. P. Putnam's Sons. 1951.
24. Bridgman, M. *Collegiate Education for Nursing.* New York: Russell Sage Foundation. 1953.
25. Throughout this section of the chapter, we have relied heavily on two publications: Anderson, O. W. *Toward an Unambiguous Profession? A Review of Nursing.* Chicago: Center for Health Administration Series, Number A6, 1968; and Davis, F. (Ed.) *The Nursing Profession.* New York: John Wiley & Sons. 1966.
26. Anderson, O. W. *Toward an Unambiguous Profession? A Review of Nursing.* Chicago: Center for Health Administration Series, Number A6, 1968. pp. 31–33.
27. American Nurses' Association., *op. cit.,* p. 15.
28. Anderson, O. W., *op. cit.,* p. 11.
29. Personal Communication from J. M. Scott, Director, Division of Nursing, Bureau of Health Manpower, accompanying a computational table dated June 5, 1967.
30. American Nurses' Association., *op. cit.,* pp. 8–9.
31. Glaser, W. A. "Nursing Leadership and Policy: Some Cross-National Comparisons." in Davis, F. (Ed.) *The Nursing Profession.* New York: John Wiley & Sons. 1966. p. 25.
32. *Ibid.*
33. *Ibid.,* pp. 25–26.
34. Anderson, O. W., *op. cit.,* p. 1.
35. *Ibid.,* pp. 1–4.
36. American Nurses' Association., *op. cit.* (Note: These figures are derived by calculations from Table 1, p. 87, and Table 3, p. 89.)
37. Davis, F., Olesen, V. L., and Whittaker, E. W. "Problems and Issues in Collegiate Nursing Education." in Davis, F. (Ed.) *The Nursing Profession.* New York: John Wiley & Sons. 1966. p. 163.
38. *Nurse Training Act of 1964. Program Review Report.* Washington, D.C.: U.S. Departmen of Health, Education, and Welfare, Public Health Service. PHS Publication No. 1740. 1967. (Note: This is commonly known as the Willard Report because of the chairmanship of Dr. W. R. Willard.)
39. American Nurses' Association., *op. cit.,* p. 14.
40. Glaser, W. A., *op. cit.,* p. 25.
41. Goldmark, J., *op. cit.,* pp. 194–195.
42. *Ibid.,* p. 195.
43. Brown, E. L., *op. cit.,* pp. 108–132. See recommendations concerning diploma schools.
44. Bridgman, M., *op. cit.,* pp. 40–70.
45. Anderson, O. W., *op. cit.,* p. 11.
46. Rogers, M. E. *Reveille in Nursing.* Philadelphia: F. A. Davis Company. 1964. p. 32.
47. *Ibid.,* p. 49.
48. American Nurses' Association., *op. cit.,* p. 106.
49. Bridgman, M., *op. cit.,* pp. 118–119.
50. *Ibid.,* p. 97.
51. Strauss, A., *op. cit.,* p. 63.
52. Davis, F., Olesen, V. L., and Whittaker, E. W., *op. cit.,* p. 168.
53. *Ibid.,* pp. 169–174.
54. Strauss, A., *op. cit.,* p. 106.

55. National League of Nursing Education. *An Activity Analysis of Nursing. A Report Prepared by the Department of Studies.* New York: National League of Nursing Education. 1932.

56. Glaser, W. A., *op. cit.,* p. 26.

57. Strauss, A., *op. cit.,* pp. 62–63.

58. Anderson, O. W., *op. cit.,* p. 36.

59. Davis, F., Olesen, V. L., and Whittaker, E. W., *op. cit.,* p. 173.

60. Strauss, A., *op. cit.,* p. 62.

61. *Ibid.*

62. Hughes, E., *et al. Twenty Thousand Nurses Tell Their Story.* Philadelphia: J. B. Lippincott Company. 1958. pp. 71–72.

63. For one example, see: Raphael, Sister Mary. "The Development and Activities of a Joint Physician-Nurse Liaison Committee," in *Report of the AMA Conference Sponsored by the AMA Committee on Nursing.* American Medical Association. 1967. p. 23.

64. American Nurses' Association., *op. cit.,* p. 74.

65. "Nursing Students Tell District No. 2 What Needs to be Done!" *Blue and White Review* Amarillo, Texas: Northwest Texas Hospital School of Nursing. 7:2:8. July, 1969.

66. Commission on Economic and General Welfare. *Reports to the House of Delegates,* 46th Convention, American Nurses' Association. New York: American Nurses' Association. 1968. pp. 74–86.

67. "Nurses Strike Los Angeles Hospital, Want C.N.A. to Bargain for Them." *Modern Hospital.* 113:1:29. July, 1969.

68. Glaser, W. A., *op. cit.,* p. 25.

69. Davis, F., Olesen, V. L., and Whittaker, E. W., *op. cit.,* p. 162.

THREE
THE CHARACTERISTICS, CONCEPTS, AND SCOPE OF NURSING PRACTICE

P rovision for full health service to the American public can be realized only when each health profession functions at its best. Thus, we must have a clear concept of the roles and functions of each profession, along with an understanding of the factors that both limit and focus the scope of its activities. In the case of nursing, we must also understand certain characteristics of nursing practice in order to deal effectively with both its basic concepts and its limitations.

CHARACTERISTICS OF NURSING PRACTICE

In the previous chapter, we examined the ways that nursing has failed, in large or small measure, to meet the common characteristics of a profession. In many respects, however, the present position of nursing results from patterns that have dominated nursing practice for several generations. Further, these conditions are so pervasive and so primary in their effect that they form, figuratively, the climates within which nurses must operate. These patterns include the nursing shortage, impoverished work environment, and role misunderstanding.

49

Climate of Nursing Shortage

Nursing has long worked in the shadow of the assumption held throughout the nation—that there is a serious, and growing, shortage of registered nurses. That there is some substance to this belief is unquestionable, but to accept it as a whole truth is harmful. Such a view about an acute shortage of nurses can lead to a coloring of all decisions about manpower development and utilization. In the case of nursing service, this is precisely what has happened.

In the section on "Needs in Relation to Fields of Nursing," the Report of the Surgeon General's Consultant Group on Nursing in 1962 had this to say:

> "A recent study of some 325 hospitals showed that about 20 percent of the positions for professional nurses were vacant, as were 18 percent of the positions for practical nurses. In New York City, over half of the positions for professional nurses in the public hospitals were unfilled in 1961. In all hospitals in Los Angeles, private as well as public, 25 to 30 percent of the positions for professional staff nurses are reported as unfilled. In a recent survey of all general hospitals in the State of Massachusetts, it was found that 20 percent of the positions for professional staff nurses were not filled."[1]

To illustrate that such a statement of facts (let us assume them to be facts) does not tell the entire story, it might be well to point out that the United States as a whole enjoyed a ratio of 298 employed professional nurses per 100,000 population in 1962. Of the three states cited above, California had 327 nurses per 100,000; New York had 388 per 100,000; and Massachusetts, no less than 514 nurses per 100,000.[2] Thus, we see that all three states had a supply of employed nurses that was above the national average. In part, the problem becomes one of "lack of fit" rather than mere "shortage."

However, the consultant group, with their strong belief in the shortage concept, projected a need for 850,000 professional nurses by 1970—a goal they felt could never be reached. They pointed out that a feasible goal of 680,000 nurses might be attained, and that this might alleviate some of the distress caused by the continuing shortage of nurses. Unless some direct, positive action were taken, however, they concluded that there would be a natural increase from 550,000 to 650,000 during the period from 1962 to 1970, and that this figure would be totally inadequate to meet the demands of the health system.[3]

Further, the consultant group identified a number of problems that stood in the way of solving the nursing shortage. These included "too few schools . . . and not enough capable young people . . . being recruited."[4] We can easily see why their recommendations incorporated assistance to schools and other health facilities in nursing education, assistance to individual students, and funds to help stimulate recruitment to schools of nursing.[5]

Of course, this was not the initial report on a nursing shortage in this country. There had been national efforts at the time of the First and Second World Wars to recruit and train large numbers of nurses, and there were a number of alarms sounded by hospital administrators and physicians before 1962. However, the eport of the consultant group focused national attention on the numbers in nurse manpower, and the public assumed that a shortage existed, or why else should there be concern.

The National Planning Association, for example, predicted a deficit in all health categories and called for an increase of 84 percent in the number of nurses, for a total of 1,091,000 by 1975.[6] The Health Manpower Commission was more modest and suggested a national goal of 900,000 nurses by 1975.[7] The Division of Nursing of the U.S. Public Health Service proposed a need for 850,000 nurses by the same year.[8] Closely related to this last number is the projection of 860,000 made by the Department of Labor.[9]

The near-magical impact of such figures causes one to consider drastic if not impetuous action to procure the needed number of nurses. Sometimes, the exhortations to meet the perceived problem sound like a clarion call to battle. In 1966, for example, Thomas Hale wrote, "There is still time to turn the tide, and the day can still be saved. But it will not happen by chance, or by letting things drift."[10] The same note of urgency has been sounded in both individual statements and resolutions adopted by such prestigious organizations as the American Nurses' Association, the American Medical Association, and the American Hospital Association.

But what is the public to think of the manpower shortage in nursing? One of the first things we should consider is how the actual supply of nurses compares with the needs projected by various expert bodies. In this regard, the outlook is not particularly distressing. For example, two analyses, one by the Department of Labor and another by the Public Health Service, had forecast a need for 620,000 and 600,000 nurses, respectively, by 1966. The actual number of active professional nurses in the United States in 1966 was 621,000.[11]

The Surgeon General's Consultant Group on Nursing forecast a need for 637,-000 nurses in 1968; the actual number of active professional nurses was 659,000. The projected need for 1970 by the same consultant group was for 680,000; the conservative estimate of our study group is that there will be approximately 695,-000 active nurses in that year.[12]

In light of these figures, the statement of the Health Manpower Commission of 1967 makes a cogent point: "In contrast to the situation for physicians and dentists, the present and projected shortages of nurses do not reflect a shortage of training facilities or of nursing graduates. . . . Given the large number of nonpracticing nurses, increasing the output of new nurses is not the best means of attacking the nurse 'shortage'."[13] In a dissent to a recommendation of the so-called Willard committee, Yett and Furstenberg comment, "However, we take exception to those aspects of the program designed to bring about a substantial increase in the quantity of professional nurses by 1975."[14]

Why are there these widely divergent views held by experts in the health field? Kissick has explained in detail that most of the projections for needed health manpower, including nursing, have been done on the basis of one of three forecasting methods: population ratios, economic projections, and professional judgment.[15] He then examines the underlying difficulties of each method.

The population ratio method, for instance, is a crude indicator that does not take into account changes in patterns of utilization and increases in productivity. Economic projections are based on a hypothesized continued expansion of total expenditures for health care at the existing rate plus an assumed expansion of effort to reduce the gap between potential and available care for all Americans. The professional judgment method relies on the projections of experts who seek ways to supply adequate to optimum care based on largely individualistic guidelines.

Perhaps the principal point of Kissick's analysis is that "the result of each of the studies cited, regardless of method employed, has been a prediction of severe shortage."[16]

Kissick goes on to say, "In discussing shortages, the focus has been on the number graduating each year. . . . As a consequence, manpower policy decisions have been related to broad assumptions of a need to increase the numbers. This is reflected in the Health Professions Educational Assistance Act of 1963, the Health Professions Education Amendments of 1965, and the Nurse Training Act of 1964, all of which aim at enlarging the manpower supply by providing financial assistance to students and funds for construction of professional schools."[17]

Relatedly, Yett has pointed out, "To date, of course, the major federal policy effort to reduce the postwar 'shortage' of nurses has not been concerned with the demand side specifically. . . . That is, even though the number of unfilled RN positions continued to be quite large, there might be no 'shortage' of nurses in terms of 'excess demand' or unmet nursing 'needs'."[18]

That there is the possibility of exaggeration in the reports on nursing shortages, and that this is not simply a matter of poor forecasting, is discussed from the viewpoint of a behavioral scientist by Glaser. "Self-interested occupations whose incomes depend on market conditions fear surpluses and prefer shortages. . . . But occupations devoted to the public service . . . usually seek more recruits and complain about shortages. . . . One of the most salient and widespread problems reported by nursing leaders throughout the world is a 'shortage' of nurses."[19]

Glaser goes on to point out, "Nursing leaders perceive shortages in countries with few graduate nurses, such as underdeveloped countries. But they also report shortages in countries where the statistics show the largest numbers of graduate nurses. For example, Great Britain and the United States. . . ."[20]

According to Glaser, there are six circumstances that govern the perceptions of shortage, real or imagined:

a. The pace of medical science which creates ever-rising demands on personnel and work pace.

b. Existence of national medical structures with personnel norms which generate feelings of shortage.

c. The creation of ideal hospital establishments and the publication of discrepancies between real and ideal.

d. Reactions to the high rate of student dropout from nursing school.

e. Reaction to the lack of commitment among graduate nurses who opt for self-interest rather than continued service in their occupation.

f. The reduction in the work week which intensifies a feeling of shortage since more nurses are needed to cover the same clock hours.[21]

Each one of these points has been evident in the discussions that have focused on nursing in the United States during the past 20 years. To the extent that Glaser is correct, student withdrawal, nurses remaining inactive, and social changes in our health system will combine with other factors to heighten the sense of shortage, even though, for example, the number of student withdrawals from nursing may be no higher than that from teaching or anthropology.

The practical effect of a continued climate of shortage is that emphasis is placed on increased supply with relatively little attention to the question of demand. The results of such policies become clear when we examine the second climate that surrounds nursing practice.

Climate of Impoverished Work Environment

To most laymen, there is an inconsistency in a situation in which a cry of shortage is persistently raised at a time when more than 285,000 individuals—almost one out of every three registered nurses—are not working in their profession.

To the same laymen, there may be two quite simplistic answers to such a problem: either train more professional nurses, or develop more auxiliaries, aides, and nonprofessionals. It may be a source of satisfaction to the general public to know that these are the very courses that have been pursued by the health specialists in this country since before 1900. It may be less satisfying to review the results.

In the first 30 years of the twentieth century, the number of nursing schools in the United States more than quadrupled—from 432 to 1,844 institutions. So rapid was the growth of these schools and the number of their graduates that the economic depression of the thirties saw widespread unemployment among nurses. In addition, nearly 500 small schools of nursing closed. The net effect of increasing the supply, without having concern for demand, was the maintenance of low salaries, long hours, and difficult schedules. As late as 1946, the Department of Labor documented the fact that nurses in the United States worked longer hours, did more night and shift work, received less overtime pay, had fewer fringe benefits, and were paid lower salaries than most workers in industry or in comparable occupational groups.[22]

During this same time, a growing number of practical nurses and nurse auxiliaries appeared on the scene. Until 1944, there were only 15 states that had licensure regulations for practical nursing, and not all of these were mandatory. The products of these training courses were of very uneven quality, but registered nurses perceived them, fairly correctly, as an economic threat. Under the exigencies of the Second World War, however, practical nursing was encouraged and given the status of a recognized vocation, and by action of the NLN's first convention in 1953, qualified practical nurses became eligible for league membership.[23]

But it is not practical nursing alone that has been tried as a solution for the nursing "shortage." Between 1967 and 1968, figures from the Willard report[24] and the *Health Resources Statistics* report of the Public Health Service[25] indicate that the number of registered nurses climbed about 3 percent, while the total of practical nurses rose almost 7 percent. In the same period, the number of aides, orderlies, and auxiliaries rose more than 14 percent to a total figure of 800,000—a group larger than the number of registered nurses, and almost as numerous as the combined total of registered and practical nurses!

The continuing role of these lower skilled and sometimes indifferently trained personnel has proceeded for many reasons, chiefly the specter of the nursing shortage. In addition, the presence of such workers helps to satisfy demands for social amelioration (that is, providing jobs for minority groups), and to provide enhancement of health careers (the auxiliary might become an aide, then a practical nurse, and perhaps even a registered nurse).

The net effect, however, has been to perpetuate what Anderson described in 1968: "In the past a large part of the servers—professional and non-professional—in the health services system were paid less than prevailing wages because of the non-profit and eleemosynary nature of health care and the dedication presumed to be expressed by the workers in being willing to care for the sick and disabled."[26]

There is a considerable body of expert opinion that challenges the traditional assumptions that the solution of the nursing shortage is to increase the supply of nurses and simultaneously expand the supply of nonprofessional aides and attendants.

Kissick has argued, "This approach of expanding the numbers, although a good and necessary beginning, has ignored the impact of the increasing applications of scientific knowledge on the delivery of health services. Health services are becoming institutionalized in a functional sense, which connotes movement from independent and isolated personal health services toward a fabric of interrelated health care services in which the individual components must be coordinated."[27] In a word, technology plus improved organization may drastically affect the need for nurses.

In their dissent to the committee report in 1967, Yett and Furstenberg are even more elemental when they state, "Without a program to translate the Nation's 'needs' into *effective* demand, the proposal to greatly increase the supply of nurses could cause large relative salary declines. Under such circumstances, nursing will become an even less attractive career than at present; and we will soon be faced with still another request for massive support to remedy the 'shortage' of nurses by increasing the supply available. This vicious circle will continue so long as market demand is below the desired goal at existing nurse salary schedules."[28]

What might happen if concern for demand operated as well as concern for supply? In his paper before the Second Conference on the Economics of Health, Yett says, "It is significant that the relatively high-salaried fields of nursing account for less than 15 percent of total R.N. employment. Moreover it is clear from both the low vacancy rates and high relative salaries that this level of employment is determined by demand."[29]

In short, if one pays a salary above the prevailing rate, then supply rises to meet demand. If this law of economics seems too simplistic as an explanation, one need only look at the events of the last six years in relation to general duty nurses. As the percentage increase in average earnings rose for those nurses, there was not only an increase in the ratio of nurses per 100,000 population, but also a larger proportion of part-time nurses who returned to practice. Thus, it would seem that the economic utility of nursing has now begun to some extent to exceed its in-utility.[30]

William H. Stewart, former Surgeon General of the United States, has said, "I think increases in nursing salaries will end up in nothing but good. If it comes to the point that the salary of a nurse makes it worthwhile for her to turn from family life back to nursing, we will attract many who have left the field. Then, too, higher salaries make nursing much more attractive as a career. And, third, it will make hospitals as well as nursing look more closely at the whole question of utilization."[31]

Of course, it is not only the lack of money that has characterized the impoverished work environment of nursing. Stewart has noted, ". . . the present situation in which nursing is caught is partly due to the problem of low salaries, poor working conditions, the increasing demands upon nurses, and changes in their functions." He goes on to observe, "Nurses are deluged with paperwork, supervision, and training duties for the many layers of assistants—practical nurses, aides and orderlies—who function between them and the people who need care."[32]

The possible effect of working through lesser trained personnel was examined by Stewart: "I cannot document this, but it seems logical that when you expand your personnel pyramid with nurses at the top, you have more and more, lesser and lesser trained people making up that pyramid, and you get to the point, what with poor quality and possible turnover, where the pyramid of personnel designed to extend the hands and skills of this professional nurse actually ends up in defeating its purpose. The result is a net loss rather than a gain."[33]

There is little doubt that low salaries, poor working conditions, and lack of professional status have led to the lack of commitment to nursing as a career, and to tangential problems in the numbers and distribution of personnel.

Climate of Role Misunderstanding

Stewart has suggested, "The hospital administrator looks at nursing in one way; the professional nurse sees it through a different pair of eyes; the physician has a different view; certainly, the patient has still another."[34]

One of the most intriguing questions that surround the controversy over nursing manpower and nursing practice relates to the role of the nurse. While this concern is examined in detail later in this chapter, and in subsequent portions of the report, it is essential that we raise a fundamental point now: The system of health care is frequently the cause for nurses leaving nursing, and it is this very system that must be modified if we are to progress toward needed changes in nursing.

We have already suggested that nurses are deluged with work that involves administration, supervision, and training, and that patient care becomes almost remote. To document this observation, we need only look at a recent analysis of the situation. The *Journal of the American Hospital Association* reported in 1969 that for the three years preceding, the ratio of nursing hours to administrative hours has steadily declined.[35] This pattern is essentially the same for hospitals of all sizes and in all regions.

Duff and Hollingshead report, "The registered nurse spent about the same amount of time in interaction with patients as physicians did. She knew comparatively little about the medical problems of patients and almost nothing about their personal problems. . . . Under these conditions, the patient and nurse could not develop a problem-solving relationship. . . ."[36]

The same authors characterize the relationship that existed as "technical, administrative, and task oriented; it was not person oriented."[37] In reporting a study on patients' thoughts about their nursing care, Ewell discovered, "In reply to a question concerning which member of the ward team provided the most frequent service, nurse's aides were mentioned most often, L.P.N.'s were next, and only 6 patients out of 76 said that the R.N. was seen most often. This probably will come as no surprise to registered nurses throughout the world who have seen their periods of direct patient contact dwindle in direct proportion to the growing nurse shortage. . . ."[38] Without repeating our concerns about the reference to the nurse "shortage," we can find helpful insights in the observations of the patients.

Suppose, for sake of argument, that a large proportion of nurses go into their field because they wish to take care of sick people. What is the situation they are likely to find in the reality of the health care system? In one analysis by Christman and Jelinek, it has been reported that "work measurement studies of nursing activities demonstrate that only about 25 to 50 percent of the skills of registered nurses are used daily. . . . *To put it another way, patients are being deprived of anywhere from 50 to 75 percent of professional nursing by this organizational format.*"[39]

Again, this is not a singular observation. At Children's Hospital in Akron, for example, a computer is now assuming a share of the tasks that have kept nurses from direct patient care. In this case, the computer calculates a daily staffing pattern for this 253-bed hospital in ten minutes, an operation that formerly took hours of nursing supervisor time.[40] It would seem that the concern over nursing involvement in non-nursing activities is justified. It would also seem that some skepticism over the nursing "shortage" may be justified, as well.

In another effort to get nurses back to nursing, Woodlawn Hospital in Chicago demonstrated that nurse utilization could ". . . be drastically improved [after] a year's experience . . . improved nurse utilization, reduced need for additional personnel, halted the rapidly rising cost of nursing service, and provided patients with more care by registered nurses."[41]

That there is satisfaction in nursing *per se* has been noted by Strauss, who comments, "Like physicians without patients, or research administrators no longer engaged in research, nurses require adequate rationales if they work away from the bedside. They require rationales not only for public legitimation of their work, but also for internal justification."[42]

The final irony, described by Yett[43] and confirmed in *Facts About Nursing,*[44] is that we tend to give status as well as monetary premiums to those nursing activities that are removed from the bedside—education and administration.

Summary of Nursing Climate

The conditions of economic depression, environmental deprivation, and role confusion are endemic to much of American nursing. To the classic economist, it may be something of a marvel that our "shortage" of nurses is not greater; certainly, many experts feel that in terms of real demand, or demand backed by money, there is no shortage at all.

Those of us who are laymen recognize that in terms of patient care needs there are, indeed, shortages of nurses, as well as all other kinds of health personnel, and that better inducements must be developed to make nursing a profitable and reinforcing career. In this regard, the two classic answers—to increase the supply of nurses and/or the supply of auxiliary workers—have proven to be failures.

CONCEPTS OF NURSING PRACTICE

Nursing has long shared with medicine a prime role in the care and treatment of the patient. While the role of the physician seems well defined, that of the nurse is far more ambiguous.[45] In fact, there appear to be three current perceptions of the nursing role that reflect basic confusions and even disagreements about the "proper" performance of a nurse.

These three concepts include the lay public's generally global view of a nurse; the occupational view of the nurse held by physicians, administrators, and some nurses; and the view of an increasing number of nurses, and some other health personnel, who regard nursing as an emerging profession. Each of these concepts alters our expectations for nursing and influences the direction that nursing practice might take in the future.

The Public Image of Nursing

To the man on the street, the nurse is a woman, dressed in white, working in a hospital, engaged in providing direct care to a patient. There may be some general awareness that there are different levels of nurses, but in all probability, the average patient would not be able to specify the varied responsibilities among those who administer care.[46]

As suggested in Figure 2, the public's view of nursing is somewhat vague and largely undifferentiated, but seen as quite separate from that of medicine. Essentially, the nurse is viewed as working in an institutional setting where an acute care problem is presented. Her efforts are directed at pain reduction, comfort, and compassionate care. To the public, the nurse is a mother-surrogate.

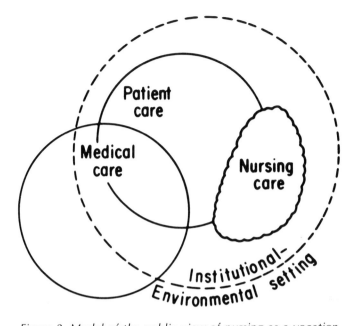

Figure 2. Model of the public view of nursing as a vocation.

Nursing, in this case, is viewed as a vocation with emphasis on such female characteristics as gentleness, consoling behavior, and pain-fear reduction. Within this context, there is little concern with quality because the entire focus is on the affective behaviors. This was dramatically illustrated in a recent study made in Illinois in which patients were asked to evaluate the adequacy of service. The subjects registered no distinctions in quality, whether care was given by registered nurses or by other categories of personnel.[47]

The impact of such a view, both on the nurse and on her role, is responsible for a number of problems. First, this public attitude toward nursing greatly restricts the recruitment of men. The public sees the nurse as "she," and this view sharply limits the attractiveness of the career for the opposite sex. Second, while the public may harbor an appreciative attitude toward the nurse, this feeling is directed toward the nurse as a person rather than as a health care professional. The public has little understanding of her education, training, or functions aside from those associated with the sickroom. This view likewise places little emphasis on formal preparation or on acceptance of the nurse as an expert.

Finally, this general attitude tends to separate nursing and medicine into distinct spheres, making certain acts appropriate when done by a physician but inappropriate when done by a nurse. Relatedly, the role of the nurse is restricted to helping activities; the public regards the doctor as the sole decision-maker on important questions of health.

Such views in our culture not only interfere with the recruitment of talented people into the profession, but also hamper the activities of those already in the nursing role. It is important to keep in mind that functions viewed as wrong for nurses in this country may be considered standard and valued practice in another cultural setting.

The Occupational View of Nursing

A second view, held by a large number of persons in health service, sees nursing as a bundle of discrete tasks designed to help and comfort patients undergoing a therapeutic program. Many physicians, administrators, and nurses find this a comfortable definition of nursing and a useful approach to the education and training of students.[48]

Figure 3 represents a model of such a view. Nursing practice is seen as functioning in acute settings and in institutional surroundings. The nurse is viewed in a

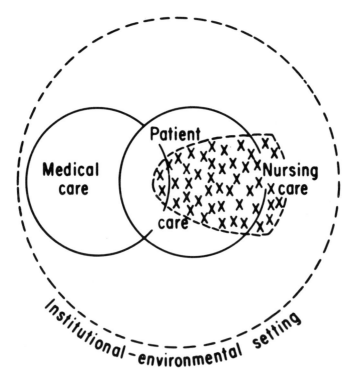

Figure 3. Model of the occupational view of nursing practice.

dependent role, carrying out the orders of the physician. Her duties consist of a large number and variety of tasks; therefore, a high premium is placed on efficiency and performance skills. While some specific treatments might be done by either the nurse or doctor on occasion, there is relatively little overlap in roles. In this model, the nurse is not seen to require much background knowledge in order to carry out her functions.[49]

As seen in this approach, the solution to providing nursing care is a simple one: train a sufficient number of hands to do the tasks. Moreover, through job analysis and time studies, it is possible that less skilled personnel may be able to perform many of these functions and thereby reduce the need for nurses. Unlike the rather amorphous view of the public toward what a nurse does, the occupational view is highly specific and task-oriented.

There are several limitations in this model. First, concentrating on the specific nursing tasks, we may conclude that more personnel will solve all patient care problems. When we look at the facts, however, we find that during a 21-year span, as Kissick reports, the ratio of nurses to patient beds changed from 1 to 15 in 1941 to 1 to 5 in 1962.[50] Yet, the nursing "shortage" continues. Another study found that patient welfare failed to improve even in face of the deliberate addition of personnel.[51] Quality would seem to be at least as important as quantity.

A second shortcoming lies in the process of planning patient care as a series of unrelated tasks performed by a variety of people. By treating nursing as primarily a body of technical functions, we tend to overlook the continuity required for patient care, and to ignore the psychosocial dimensions of treatment and recovery. As Duff and Hollingshead suggest, there are factors involved in patient care that lie outside the province of task analysis; yet these have a commanding influence on the course of a patient's progress and recovery. Lack of total patient care can produce a disability as great as any caused by disease.[52]

Finally, this occupational view of nursing has inhibited the development of an intellectual approach to role performance and has caused an imbalance in the entire health services system. As indicated in Figure 4, the assumption of task boundaries for nursing and other health occupations has caused the development of a grotesque educational pyramid, in which highly educated and skilled physicians are expected to work through a vast number of less skilled and less educated persons. As one can see, the second foundation of the structure consists of nurses who are separated by a wider gulf from the physician than they are from the attendants and aides. This disparity hampers the efforts to both recruit and retain competent individuals. To the extent that Maslow and other motivational psychologists are correct, we could anticipate that nurses would wish to develop their intellect as well as their capacity to serve, and that the most intelligent will chafe at this task approach.[54]

Years Post—high School Education   Illustrative Occupations

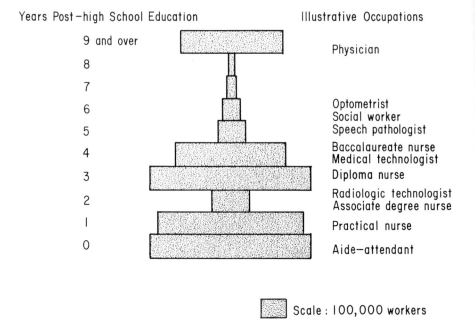

Figure 4. *The medical services pyramid.* [53]

Nursing as an Emerging Professional Practice

A third concept of nursing, depicted in Figure 5, has been urged primarily by organized nursing groups and their leaders. It focuses on the intellectual demands placed on the nurse, and emphasizes the growth in her decision-making responsibilities. While it designates a separate domain of expertise and practice, this approach sees nursing as a team effort interacting with the physician and other health workers.

In addition, this model is much less bound by the institutional setting. It sees the nurse engaged in the community as well as in the hospital or nursing home. It sees nursing practice separated into professional and technical components, with education as the entree to both, but with added knowledge required for professional decision-making and leadership.

This approach to nursing practice stems from increased study of the behavioral sciences. It also represents a determined effort by the profession to develop a science of nursing that will permit accurate prediction and control of the outcomes of nursing intervention.

With its emphasis on intellectual growth and stimulation, this approach would seem to hold promise for the profession. However, there are some distinct drawbacks.

Perhaps the most controversial aspect is the separation of the nursing role into professional and technical components. The possible result would be to remove the best prepared individuals from patient care, and place less emphasis on actual nursing practice. In such a case, the profession would be repeating some of the past practices that tended to take nurses from the patient and place them in managerial roles.[55] In all likelihood, this drawback stems in part from a semantic problem; professional practice always incorporates elements of technical skill. McDowell, for example, found that the best qualified nurses perform a variety of technical tasks as they provide patient care.[56] The semantic overtone is unfortunate; however, it could be modified easily.

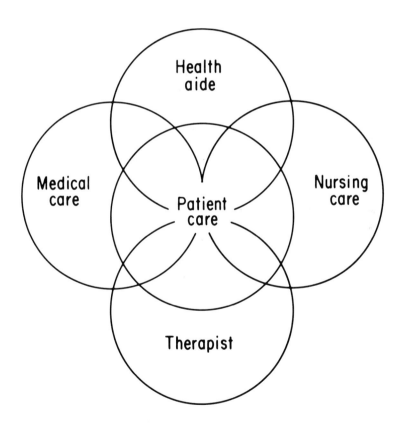

Figure 5. Model of the emergent view of nursing as a profession.

A second shortcoming stems from the intense focus on the psychosocial dimensions of nursing care, so that the physical sciences, as factors in nursing practice, are in danger of neglect. One obvious consequence is that most of the recent research in the field of nursing reflects the psychosocial concern, and almost no physiologically based studies have been reported.[57]

Finally, in its effort to document a separate realm for nursing, this current view of nursing's role tends to exaggerate its distinctions from medical care. This is contrary to the profession's own emphasis on team practice, and may simply reinforce the separatist occupational view harbored by medicine and administration toward nursing.

Impact of the Rival Perceptions

In the final analysis, each of these views of the nursing role contains some elements of value, and some that are not very valuable. The general, or lay, view of nursing endorses the social importance of the profession. The occupational view emphasizes the technical competence and skill level of the nurse practitioner. The professional view adds the dimensions of thinking and judgment to produce a whole nurse.

If nursing is to develop its role to gain widespread endorsement of its aims, then it must recognize both the nurturing needs of the public and the technical requirements of the other health associates, and somehow blend these into the development of the new nurse—a professional practitioner.

SCOPE OF NURSING PRACTICE

Development of the advanced scope of nursing practice should incorporate the best elements of the three current views of the profession: a keen sensitivity to the patient's wants, a comprehensive knowledge of procedures and technology, and a clear grasp of the behavioral and physical sciences that provide a basis for judgment.

To clarify the scope of nursing practice, both as it is today and as it will be, we have built a conceptual model through which we can describe and analyze current practice, as well as project the characteristics that seem likely to grow out of the current thrust in health care delivery.

A Model of Nursing Practice

This conceptual model is based on an in-depth study of literature in the health field, including a review of more than 900 reports on the utilization of nurses and related personnel in patient care. But even more important, it is shaped by over 100 on-site visits throughout the United States, plus related interviews and surveys. These personal observations took place in all the settings where nurses may be found: hospitals, clinics, industrial plants, educational institutions, and public health agencies. From the ensuing discussions with more than 1,000 nurses, physicians, administrators, researchers, students, and consumers, we have attempted to construct a logical representation of the domain of nursing practice.

Certainly, the process of applying analysis to nursing is not original; in most ways, the characterization that we have drawn is consistent with the findings of other observers of the health care field.[58] From the literature, from observed behavior, and from expert opinion, it would seem that nursing might be described on the basis of a three-dimensional figure—a cube that permits us to assign spatial entity to practice while simultaneously considering three key variables. These variables, which are represented by the three dimensions of the cube, are specific

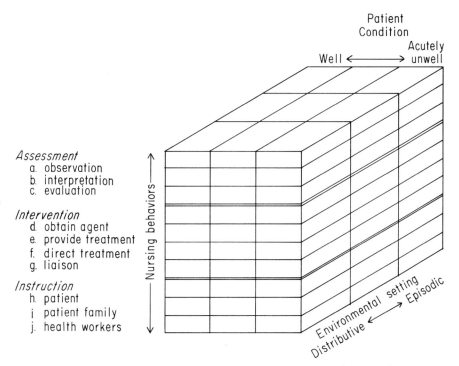

Figure 6. *Interactive model of three variables in nursing practice: nursing behaviors, patient condition, and environmental setting.*

nursing behaviors, the condition of the patient, and the environmental setting in which care takes place. Figure 6 illustrates the dynamic relationships that obtain in the model.

Ranged along the vertical dimension of the cube are the primary tasks of nursing. Subdivided into three categories, these include the elements of assessment, intervention, and instruction. In current nursing situations, these activities encompass both simple and highly complex functions, many of which are outside the purview of either the public or the occupational concepts of nursing.

The observation process, for example, includes the traditional tasks of taking and recording vital signs of pulse and temperature. In addition, however, this activity encompasses such complexities as monitoring cardiac changes, taking an entire patient history, and performing complete physical examinations.[59] Interpretation occurs when the nurse translates inferences about patient care into concrete action. The spectrum ranges from such a simple situation as needed patient rest to the construction of a complex plan for care as required by the Joint Commission on Hospital Accreditation.[60] The evaluation process includes assessing the results of treatment, auditing patient responses, and setting priorities for care.[61]

While most of the functions associated with assessment are obscured by the more visible aspects of nursing performance, their accuracy and quality are crucial for effective patient care and for the capacity of the health system to respond to new requirements for the delivery of adequate care. The vignette of a nurse specialist in cardiac therapy, observing and interpreting the responses of a patient in an intensive care unit, might be symbolic of the extent to which individual nurses become responsible for fundamental decisions.

More customary, certainly, in the public view of nursing, are the activities included under the title of intervention. At the lowest skill levels, these tasks can consist of summoning the house doctor, making a bed, calling an aide for assistance, or discussing a patient with a therapist. Such behaviors can be categorized, broadly, as follows: obtain agent, provide treatment, direct treatment, and act as liaison personnel. However, the needs of the health system, plus the changing demands on nursing, document the fact that these are foundation behaviors that must be viewed in balance with highly sophisticated forms of intervention.

The nurse in the cardiac unit, for example, is exhibiting another level of these skills, ranged across the category headings. When she alerts the cardiologist to a change in the patient's status and simultaneously moves to apply defibrillator paddles, this nurse is leading a team of auxiliaries trained to provide quick response and errorless performance.[62] In terms of liaison activity, nurses may be found today leading others in the search for solutions to health related problems that involve social workers, prosthetic fabricators, welfare counsels, and health aides.[63] Essentially, the nurse can be involved in judgment and decision-making on a level not envisioned in the traditional view of nursing. Most observers agree, too, that this trend is both growing and accelerating. Today's concept of nursing practice must include these higher reaches of clinical intervention.

The third category, instruction, is so common that it is often overlooked in the rush of day-to-day activities. From the instruction of expectant mothers to the specialized teaching of diabetic patients, nurses have continually enlarged both the scope and the quality of their educating roles.[64] As Medicaid and Medicare bring more elderly and impoverished persons into the purview of the health system, it has become apparent that nurses must develop courses and informal training sessions for families of patients, as well as lead seminars and workshops for health workers of every description.[65]

Equally cogent as a variable is the range of conditions found in persons needing care, assessment, and instruction. In both the general and occupational views of nursing, primary emphasis is on the care of the acute patient. These approaches hold that nurses properly interact with patients in extreme condition. There are those who insist, however, that nursing and the other health professions will never begin their essential service until they move in the direction of health maintenance and disease prevention, rather than maintain the almost defensive posture of assisting in cure and recuperation.[66]

In our model of nursing practice, we have attempted to visualize a variety of nursing roles, with service to individuals who range from the well to the acutely unwell. The pediatric nurse practitioner, for example, may see many children who are well, and counsel their parents in ways to see that they stay healthy.[67] In another situation, the nurse specialist may be functioning in an ambulatory care clinic where she is working essentially with patients having chronic or debilitating illnesses. She may not see healthy patients, but her work does focus on those who are mildly ill, and her role is influenced by their needs.[68] It is true that the majority of nurses today are engaged in the time-honored tasks of aiding the seriously ill. Although almost two-thirds of our nurses work in the hospital setting,[69] we should not overlook the importance—the vitality—of nursing activity that can minimize or even prevent the factors that result in hospital admissions. In any event, we need to recognize and analyze the roles of nurses concerned with patients other than the acutely unwell.

The third conditioning factor in the scope of nursing practice is the environmental setting. Just as any social organization develops its *mores* and *taboos,* so the social environment associated with the provision of health care strongly influences its conduct, and its results. Because of the fundamental induction of nurses into the hospital setting, we have frequently overlooked the requirements for nursing in the distributive, rather than the episodic, context. For instance, the professional conduct of a nurse in a ghetto neighborhood clinic is bound by different guidelines from those of a nurse in the acute ward of a general hospital. Not only are the patients different in their needs, but the very approach of the nurse to her role will shift within such disparate settings.[70]

The largest readjustment in our health care system must come in the channeling of comprehensive care to entire segments of our population that do not receive it now. Of necessity, this aid must recognize the cultural and environmental differences that influence even the acceptance or rejection of help. While we do not plead for a reduction in emphasis on hospital nursing, we can project, through an analysis of nursing requirements, that the amount of distributive nursing will have to increase markedly in the future. Professionals must be trained to function effectively in surroundings and situations that are unusual, if not unique, in our present health delivery organization.[71]

When we examine among these three factors—behaviors, settings, and patient conditions—we can begin to predict the future role of the nurse practitioner. The following notations describing a single episode in the treatment of a tubercular patient illustrate the changing scope of nursing practice:

> "Following the initial investigation, in which it was determined that the tuberculosis infection was inactive, a more vigorous attempt was made to educate the patient. . . . In these areas, the nursing team was chiefly active, with the physician occupying a supervisory and supportive role.
>
> "Plans were made. . . . Evaluation of the patient's understanding . . . showed . . . an educational program was needed to ensure a minimally adequate diet. . . . Follow-up examinations and support were arranged, with the assistance of public health nursing services.
>
> "Physical therapy activities were supervised and carefully taught in the home. . . . This goal called for a degree of preventive health care exceeding that which would be given in a custodial situation."[72]

The preceding statements were quoted at some length because they contain elements of our entire conceptual model: varied nursing patterns in response to changing patient conditions and a changing locus for treatment. We must point out that the patient and the nursing team remained the same human beings throughout the course of therapy, but their relationship and tasks were flexible in response to the total situation.

The conceptual model, then, permits us to visualize the diversity of activities that can best be described by the multiple cells in the cube of practice. Further, it allows us to illustrate what happens when nursing functions are modified in connection with patient condition and/or environmental settings. It is hoped that it also offers us an analytical construct for predicting and controlling major elements of nursing in terms of the scope and conditions for practice. In that light, it can help us foresee the numbers of nurses who must be equipped to meet the changing needs of society in the coming years.

The Changing Scope of Nursing Practice

It would be wasted effort to develop a conceptual model for nursing if its purpose were simply one of academic exercise, unrelated to the real world of need and process. In at least three important areas, our model suggests vectors of change that will affect the basic directions of the nursing profession. In the examination of the data arranged within the cells, there emerges a pictorial indication of what the next few years will hold: striking changes in the levels of nursing; greater development of clinical specialization; and significant alterations in the reciprocal roles held by nurses and other health personnel, particularly the physician. While each of these shifts in the scope of nursing practice reflects the interplay of the three-dimensional variables in the model, it can be shown that each of the projected changes in practice is associated primarily with one of the major constructs of the model.

The anticipated *changes in the levels of nursing practice,* for example, will interact most clearly with the dimension of *nursing behavior.* In contrast to the fairly limited practices of the past (see Figure 6), which emphasized the observation (temperature, pulse, and respiration) and treatment (passing of medications) tasks, we can now project a great diversification in the nursing role. In all the categories of assessment, for example, the combination of technology and research permits the nurse to effectively monitor the essential factors that contribute to patient care. Today, by evaluating the readings of sophisticated equipment, a nurse can gather better information, in both quality and quantity, on the state of a cardiac patient than a cardiologist could have done 15 years ago.[73]

Similarly, there is a great difference in the treatment of ambulatory patients as provided by the nurse of ten years ago when compared to the practices that can be observed today and those that can be projected for tomorrow. Nurses in one experimental study, for example, conducted physical examinations, prescribed drugs, ordered laboratory tests, reviewed treatment and problems, and generally assumed major responsibility for the treatment of patients.[74]

Emphasis on instruction has grown with our recognition of the increased need for nationwide preventive health care and maintenance. The greatest single area of growth within the several categories of nursing specialty is that of the school nurse.[75] An increasing number of public and occupational health nurses are directing their efforts toward teaching better health maintenance practices to individuals and selected target groups. Relatedly, there is a growing awareness of the need for improved in-service education of health personnel, and the critical role that nurses must play in this form of instruction.[76]

Just as the changing levels of nursing practice relate to the increased dimension of the nursing role, so the projected *change toward clinical specialization* is related to the *condition of the patient*. Traditionally, nursing has been directed to care of the acutely ill. The concepts of public health nursing, while valued, have not enjoyed the emphasis of the functions for acute episodic care.

Peplau has drawn a picture of clinical specialization in transition. She suggests a broad diversification in future nursing practice that will encompass far more work with the well person along with the chronic or debilitated patient who would not be described as acutely unwell.[77] In addition, a growing number of specialists, such as those working in burn therapy, are showing a pattern of practice quite similar to that of medicine; they are on call in the event that a severely burned patient is admitted. Then they remain with the patient through treatment, recovery, rehabilitation, and readjustment.[78] In such a specialty, the nurse clinician handles all degrees of patient condition and encompasses all aspects of functional nursing behavior.

The importance of this growing trend toward clinical specialization can hardly be overstated. Despite the somewhat disorganized appearance of the present state of affairs, with a lack of agreement on what the fields of specialty should be and what constitutes the core knowledge within a specialty, the nurse clinician is the best hope to fill the professional gap in the health care system. Through this approach, nursing can provide a solution to the known shortcomings of a health system in which one out of four persons is receiving less than adequate care. If nursing can contribute, also, to the upgrading of care for the other 75 percent of our population, its growing clinical capacity to serve, and its greater service to the well and those who are not acutely ill will probably provide this capability. At the same time, the profession must continue to serve in the episodic facilities for those individuals who need nursing care most critically.

The third anticipated change in the scope of nursing practice relates to *alterations in the reciprocal roles of the nurse and the physician*. While this change will be reflected in the model through nursing behavior and patient conditions, it will be focused primarily in terms of the *environmental setting* (see Figure 6) in which nursing functions are provided.

Along with many other writers in the field, Duff and Hollingshead call for the development of a medical auxiliary to fill the known gaps in the health care delivery system.[79] To staff this area, programs have been established to train "physicians' assistants" whose functions would be carried out in the present void (see Figure 4) that exists between the doctor and the nurse.[80]

In contrast to the development of a new specialty and a new corps of health workers, there is a simultaneous movement toward increased clinical specialization in nursing. This approach is aimed at many of the same objectives: enhanced patient care, extension of care to more individuals, and better professional distribution of functional tasks. However, the unique identity of the nurse as a professional practitioner is maintained.

There is some feeling that this latter approach may be more effective in reaching the objectives. Former Surgeon General Stewart, for one, describes the essential relationship of medicine and nursing in this way: "Medicine is a profession, rooted in science. Its practice is the application of scientific knowledge which can become an art. . . . Nursing is the same; it is a profession, not a science in and of itself. Like medicine, it has deep roots in science, and as science advances, the roots go deeper."[81]

Given this fundamental agreement in approach, it would seem that the best use of today's nurses (the largest and one of the most highly qualified groups of health professionals) would lie in the extension of their activities to meet society's needs. Actually, the trend toward better role articulation for health care professionals has already been identified. Now, the question is one of how the changed relationships can best be fully evolved.[82]

The most effective development of reciprocal roles between nurse and physician can be seen in research studies aimed at defining specialized functions in terms of patient need rather than through *a priori* assumptions of proper spheres of nursing and medical practice.[83] The results of one such effort have been documented in a case in which physicians and nurses were involved in ambulatory patient care (see Figure 7).[84]

An analysis of reciprocal health roles in nursing and medicine confirms that nurses are sharing more and more activities with the physician. This development is even more pronounced in the emerging institutional settings created to narrow the gap between actual and optimal health care. In group practice, neighborhood clinics, visiting nurse services, and extended care facilities, nurses are often called on to exercise the qualities of clinical specialization and practice.

With these changes, however, there must come alterations in organizational structures and expectations along the entire dimension of environmental setting (see Figure 6). In the established regimen of the hospital, it may come as a surprise that many nurses wish to function in patient care, and resist serving as pharmacists and other health workers during various hours of the day or night. It will come as a definite shock that some nurses insist on a definition of their profession that is closer to that of medicine than the traditional one of the hospital nurse. For example, the practice of a nurse being on call is established in a few, but only a

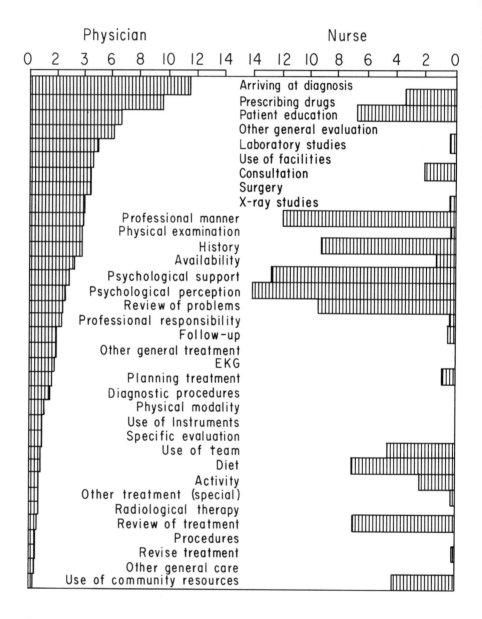

Figure 7. Representation of nurse and physician relationships in a dynamic setting.

few, hospitals. The role of the pediatric nurse-practitioner is operational in only a limited number of settings at present. The trend is unmistakable, however, and positive efforts should be aimed at revamping the traditional organizational patterns to keep up with the expanding scope of nursing practices.

The choice before the institutions and organizations involved in health care is clear: Will they anticipate and adjust their operations in accordance with changed requirements of today's society, or will they continue with the *status quo* knowing that our current system is already incapable of meeting the needs of the country.

In summary, three discernible trends emerge from our analysis of nursing practice: diversification of the levels of nursing practice; increased development of clinical nursing specialization; and restructuring of the traditional relationships between nursing and medicine. These trends, separately and in combination, will have a profound effect on the scope of future nursing practice, making it more professional, more scientific, and far more meaningful to the entire health care system of the United States.

Effects of Nursing Practice

Despite the national concern over the "shortage" of nurses, and some of the disagreements that exist about the nursing role, there is a general lack of knowledge about the outcome of nursing practice. In contrast to the dramatic results of surgical intervention, the efforts of a nurse are less conspicuous, and are quite likely to be overlooked in the welter of activities that go on in most health care settings. Everyone "knows" that nurses are vital to health processes, but the general and occupational views of nursing scarcely look on nursing care as crucial to the outcome of treatment.

In the past decade, just as the scope of nursing practice has become influenced by a variety of factors, so we have seen research data that describe and explain the outcomes of nursing behavior. The findings are truly significant because they document the fact that quality nursing care can (a) improve the actual treatment accorded the patient; (b) improve the economics connected with the delivery of health care; and (c) provide the personal reinforcement needed by the nurses themselves to deepen their commitment to the field.

In terms of the improvement in actual patient care, there is more and more evidence that nursing can contribute meaningfully to better treatment and safer therapy. As research into the profession goes deeper, a number of findings attest to the benefits of quality nursing. For example, one investigation demonstrated that procedures executed by highly trained practitioners in using Foley catheters significantly decreased the incidence of infection and illness. The most profound thing about this particular study, perhaps, is that it was conducted *by nurses* and was concerned with *nursing behaviors.* Another investigation sought to establish the relationship between expert nursing prior to surgery (in order to reduce preoperative stress) and the speed of patient recovery. A significant positive relationship was found. In still a third project, quality nursing care resulted in the elimination of decubitus ulcers and other difficulties associated with extended periods of patient immobility.[85] All these findings seem congruent with our general expectations; yet they go beyond the surface conclusion and define the variables that obtain in a particular situation and in the dimensions of nursing care that can significantly affect patient recovery.

In yet another demonstration, the impact of intensive postsurgery nursing plans was subjected to controlled analysis. The results showed that patients receiving the experimental nursing care had one-fifth the untoward reactions that were experienced by the control patients receiving conventional care.[86] Finally, another study of patient energy expenditures before and after surgery led to provision of a modified system of ambulation activities to speed recovery.[87]

This brief survey of a small portion of the literature is suggestive of the growing efforts to develop research capabilities and to apply the findings to the improvement of patient care. Increasingly, hard data have been accumulated that attest to the effects of nursing practice.

In face of burgeoning costs throughout the health system, it is important to recognize that the scope of nursing practice can have an important effect on the economics of patient care. Earlier, we reported the results of inquiries into the organization of nursing service. Some observers have suggested that by freeing nurses to do nursing, patients might have access to 50 to 75 percent more care, without any increase in the number of practitioners.[88] In one instance, the establishment of a centralized patient transport service, nursing time increased by 560 hours each week for direct patient care.[89] Proper utilization of nurses, then, can contribute to real savings in personnel and attendant costs.

There is growing evidence that nursing can make other contributions to the improvement of health economics, as well. One study has demonstrated that improved nursing management of the chronically ill can reduce the number of required patient visits and still provide better follow-up in their cases.[90] Still another careful analysis of ambulatory patient care disclosed that better nursing practice could halve the staff time required to care for the individuals and yet materially reduce patient waiting time.[91]

Speed patient recovery, reduce the staff of professionals and auxiliaries through better procedures, and conserve the time of physicians by encouraging nurses to function at their highest capacities—these are the major economic benefits that can be realized. In face of the problems now confronting our health care system, the contribution of nursing service may be our best hope for keeping costs within any set of controls.

Finally, enhanced nursing practice, as a rewarding day-to-day activity itself, can lead to the continuation of nurses in direct patient care and contact. Recognizing this thrust in the changing scope of practice, the American Nurses' Association Commission on Nursing Education recently made the following statement:

> "The major purpose of graduate study in nursing should be the preparation of nurse clinicians capable of improving nursing care through the advancement of nursing theory and science."[92]

Analyzing what has happened in the past, the commission admits that there have been errors:

> "Traditionally, graduate education in nursing has been considered as preparation for particular functions and positions—primarily, teaching and administration. This emphasis, unfortunately, has tended to devalue nursing care and practice, by suggesting that there is no more to nursing knowledge than can be encompassed in the initial, undergraduate preparation."[93]

Many of the rewards within nursing have been those that drew nurses out of patient care; now, the professional organization is attempting to shift directions. The effort to enhance nursing practice has also been supported by those physicians, administrators, and other health personnel who want to see an extension in the role of the nurse clinician. We believe that this is the direction of future practice and we urge that nursing roles be recast in terms of the obvious currents in our culture and the health needs of the American public.

SUMMARY

Nursing practice has long operated under unfavorable conditions. The general assumption of a nursing shortage and the short-term solutions to that problem have resulted in unwise utilization of personnel and diminished nursing quality. Likewise, the generally impoverished work environment of nursing has offered little inducement to professional commitment, long careers, or prolonged preparation for highly specialized nursing practice. Finally, the general confusion over the proper role of nursing has led alternately to global or task-specific formulations. One view makes nursing indescribable and the other relegates it to such particularized functions that it seems like a technical vocation rather than a professional endeavor.

The general, occupational, and emerging professional approaches to the role of nursing contain much that is true and worthwhile. However, each is inadequate to meet the full range of patient needs. Rather than formulate a series of practices or standards that purport to encompass nursing, we have attempted to construct a conceptual model. This approach is based on three variables (nursing behaviors, patient condition, and environmental setting) that permit us to locate and describe all nursing activities in the configuration of a cube. From this model, we can trace nursing practice as it exists today and project important trends for the future.

Three movements are occurring in nursing practice today that will influence future patterns:

—Levels of nursing practice are becoming more diversified.
—The clinical specialist is emerging as a new professional.
—The reciprocal roles of nurses and physicians are undergoing basic changes.

In each instance, we see the necessity for better research, better preparation, better opportunities, and better rewards for nursing practice—in order to keep the nurse engaged in direct patient care.

Finally, we have looked at the evidence that shows how the current and projected changes in the scope of nursing practice can provide higher levels of quality patient care, improved economics in health facilities, and more interesting day-to-day activities that will reinforce a nurse's commitment to remain in the field of patient care. The net effect could be greater professionalism, a stronger commitment to nursing itself, and longer career lives.

The goal of nursing, as well as other health professions, should be to facilitate these changes in order to move with society toward the solution of our recurrent health problems.

FOOTNOTES

1. *Toward Quality in Nursing.* Report of the Surgeon General's Consultant Group on Nursing. Washington, D.C.: U.S. Department of Health, Education, and Welfare, Public Health Service. PHS Publication No. 992. 1963. p. 15.
2. American Nurses' Association. *Facts About Nursing, 1967 Edition.* New York: American Nurses' Association. 1967. p. 13.
3. *Toward Quality in Nursing., op. cit.,* pp. 21, 54. (With reference to projected needs it is interesting to note that the Division of Nursing reports 680,000 registered nurses, including part-time, in practice as of January 1, 1969.)
4. *Ibid.,* p. 5.
5. *Ibid.,* pp. 56–57.

6. Lecht, Leonard A. *Manpower Needs for National Goals in the 1970's.* New York: Frederick A. Praeger. 1969. p. 147.

7. *Report of the National Advisory Commission on Health Manpower, Volume I.* Washington, D.C.: U.S. Government Printing Office. 1967. p. 22.

8. *Health Manpower Source Book. Section 2. Nursing Personnel.* Revised January 1966. Washington, D.C.: U.S. Department of Health, Education, and Welfare, Public Health Service. PHS Publication No. 263. 1966. p. 108.

9. *Health Manpower 1966-75. A Study of Requirements and Supply.* Washington, D.C.: U.S. Department of Labor, Bureau of Labor Statistics. Report No. 323. 1967. p. 23.

10. Hale, T. "Problems of Supply and Demand in the Education of Nurses." *The New England Journal of Medicine.* 275:19:1048. November 10, 1966.

11. American Nurses' Association. *Facts About Nursing, 1968 Edition.* New York: American Nurses' Association. 1968. p. 10.

12. This figure is obtained by a downward rounding of a straight line projection based on the actual change in numbers of active registered nurses over the period 1962 through 1968. Without rounding, the figure is actually over 697,000 nurses that might be expected to be active in 1970.

13. *Report of the National Advisory Commission on Health Manpower, Volume I, op. cit.,* pp. 22-23.

14. *Nurse Training Act of 1964. Program Review Report.* Washington, D.C.: U.S. Department of Health, Education, and Welfare, Public Health Service. PHS Publication No. 1740. 1967. p. 3.

15. Kissick, W. L. "Forecasting Health Manpower Needs: The 'Numbers Game' Is Obsolete." *Hospitals.* 41:18:47. September 16, 1967. p. 49.

16. *Ibid.,* p. 51.

17. *Ibid.*

18. Yett, D. E. "Yes, Virginia, There Is a Shortage of Nurses—But, It's Not Quite as Simple as All That. . . ." Paper delivered at the Second Conference on the Economics of Health: Baltimore, Maryland, December 5-7, 1968., *mimeo.,* p. 67.

19. Glaser, W. A. "Nursing Leadership and Policy: Some Cross-National Comparisons." in Davis, F. (Ed.) *The Nursing Profession.* New York: John Wiley & Sons. 1966. p. 31.

20. *Ibid.,* p. 32.

21. *Ibid.,* pp. 33-36.

22. Bullough, V. L. and Bullough, B. *The Emergence of Modern Nursing, Second Edition.* New York: The Macmillan Company. 1969. p. 227.

23. Jensen, D. M. *History and Trends in Professional Nursing, Fourth Edition.* St. Louis, Missouri: C. V. Mosby Company. 1959. p. 321.

24. *Nurse Training Act of 1964. Program Review Report., op. cit.,* p. 55.

25. *Health Resources Statistics.* Report from the National Center for Health Statistics. Washington, D.C.: U.S. Department of Health, Education, and Welfare, Public Health Service. PHS publication No. 1509. 1968. pp. 135-137.

26. Anderson, O. W. *Toward an Unambiguous Profession? A Review of Nursing.* Chicago: Center for Health Administration Series, Number A6, 1968. p. 1.

27. Kissick, W. L., *op. cit.,* p. 51.

28. *Nurse Training Act of 1964. Program Review Report., op. cit.,* p. 3.

29. Yett, D. E., *op. cit.,* p. 38.

30. American Nurses' Association. *supra.,* pp. 132 and 7-10.

31. "The Surgeon General Looks at Nursing." *American Journal of Nursing.* 67:1:66. January, 1967.

32. *Ibid.,* p. 65.

33. *Ibid.*

34. *Ibid.*

35. "Administrative Profiles." *Hospitals.* 43:8:26. April 16, 1969.

36. Duff, R. S. and Hollingshead, A. B. *Sickness and Society.* New York: Harper & Row. 1968. p. 374.

37. *Ibid.*

38. Ewell, C. M., Jr. "What Patients Really Think about Their Nursing Care." *Modern Hospital.* 109:6:107. December, 1967.

39. Christman, L. P. and Jelinek, R. C. "Old Patterns Waste Half the Nursing Hours." *Modern Hospital.* 108:1:79. January, 1967.

40. DeMarco, James P. and Snavely, Shirley A. "Nurse Staffing with a Data Processing System." *American Journal of Nursing.* 63:10:122-125. October, 1963.

41. Jacobs, D. J. "Position Control Plan Slows Rise in Cost of Nursing Service." *Hospitals.* 41:11:73. June 1, 1967.

42. Strauss, A. "The Structure and Ideology of American Nursing: An Interpretation." in Davis, F. (Ed.) *The Nursing Profession.* New York: John Wiley & Sons. 1966. p. 96.

43. Yett, D. E., *op. cit.,* p. 38.

44. American Nurses' Association. *supra.,* pp. 127–159. See also, *Survey of Salaries of Teaching and Administrative Personnel in Nursing Educational Programs, September, 1968.* New York: American Nurses' Association, Research and Statistics Department, Publication No. D-35. 1969.

45. Anderson, O. W., *op. cit., passim.*

46. Hughes, E., *et al. Twenty Thousand Nurses Tell Their Story.* Philadelphia: J. B. Lippincott Company. 1958. pp. 199 and 206.

47. Levine, E. *Study of Factors Affecting the Utilization of Nursing Personnel in 31 Hospitals in Illinois.* Author's manuscript prepublication draft. 1969. p. 43.

48. Pellegrino, E. "The Physician and the Nurse." *Annals of Internal Medicine.* 64:5:1140. May, 1966. Hale, T. "Cliches of Nursing Education." *The New England Journal of Medicine.* 278:16:879, 886. April 18, 1968.

49. Hale, T. "Cliches of Nursing Education." *op. cit.,* pp. 881–882.

50. Kissick, W. "Health Manpower in Transition." *The Milbank Memorial Fund Quarterly.* 41:Part 2:59. January, 1968.

51. Aydelotte, M. and Tenner, M. *An Investigation of the Relation Between Nursing Activity and Patient Welfare.* Iowa City, Iowa: State University of Iowa. 1960.

52. Duff, R. S. and Hollingshead, A. B., *op. cit.,* pp. 123, 178, 213, 299, 377, *passim.*

53. *Health Manpower Perspective: 1967.* U.S. Public Health Service Publication No. 1677. Washington, D.C.: U.S. Government Printing Office. 1967. p. 17.

54. Maslow, A. *Motivation and Personality.* New York: Harper & Bros. 1954. See the continuum of motivational needs at the psychosocial level.

55. Christman, L. "Specialism and Generalism in Clinical Nursing." *Hospitals.* 41:1:83. January 1, 1967. Meyer, G. *Tenderness and Technique: Nursing Values in Transition.* Institute of Industrial Relations, University of California at Los Angeles, Monograph Series No. 6. Los Angeles: University of California. 1960. pp. 6–7.

56. McDowell, W. "Nurse-Patient-Physician Behavior: Nursing Care and the Regulation of Patient Condition." *The Nurse-Patient-Doctor Triadic Relationships: Effects on Nursing Care of the Patient.* New York: American Nurses' Association. 1962. pp. 18–29.

57. Schlotfeldt, R., *et al.* "Research—How Will Nursing Define It?" *Nursing Research.* 16:2:108-129. Spring, 1967. See also series of articles in *Nursing Research.* 17:3.

May–June, 1968; 17:5. September–October, 1968; 17:6. November–December, 1968. U.S. Department of Health, Education, and Welfare, Public Health Service, Division of Nursing. *Current Nursing Research Grants.* PHS Publication No. 1762. 1968.

58. Abdellah, F. G., Beland, I. L., Martin, A., and Matheny, R. V. *Patient Centered Approaches to Nursing.* New York: The Macmillan Company. 1960. Beland, I. L. *Clinical Nursing.* New York: The Macmillan Company. 1965. Henderson, V. *The Nature of Nursing.* New York: The Macmillan Company. 1966. Kron, F. *Nursing Team Leadership. Second Edition.* Philadelphia: W. B. Saunders Company. 1966. Reiter, F. and Kakosh, M. *Quality of Nursing Care—A Report of a Field Study to Establish Criteria,* conducted at the Division of Nursing Education, Teachers College, Columbia University, 1950–1954. New York: Graduate School of Nursing, New York Medical College. 1963. Rinehart, E. L. *Management of Nursing Care.* New York: The Macmillan Company. 1969. Yura, H. and Walsh, M. B. *The Nursing Process.* Washington, D.C.: Catholic University of America Press. 1967.

59. Ford, L. C. and Silver, H. K. "The Expanded Role of the Nurse in Child Care." *Nursing Outlook.* 15:9:44. September, 1967. Lewis, C. E. *The Dynamics of Nursing in Ambulatory Patient Care.* U.S. Public Health Service Grant No. NU-00145 Final Report. Author's manuscript. pp. 18–22. Rinehart, E. L., *op. cit.,* pp. 1–33. Yura, H. and Walsh, M. B., *op. cit.,* pp. 1–43.

60. Henderson, V. *The Nature of Nursing, op. cit.,* pp. 28–29. Johnson, M. "Joint Commission on the Accreditation of Hospitals." *Nursing Outlook.* 6:5:258. May 1958. Rinehart, E. L., *op. cit.,* pp. 129–153. Yura, H. and Walsh, M. B., *op. cit.,* pp. 44–95.

61. Yura, H. and Walsh, M. B., *op. cit.,* pp. 95–108.

62. Rinehart, E. L., *op. cit.,* pp. 98–121.

63. Interview, New York-Cornell Hospital, 5/2/69; interview, Tufts University Columbia Point Health Center, Boston, Massachusetts, 2/20/69; interview, Visiting Nurse Association of New York, 4/29/69.

64. Hommel, F., Florence, H., and Estey, G. Series of articles on "Natural Childbirth." *American Journal of Nursing.* 69:7:1446–1453. July, 1969. Scahill, M. "Preparing Children for Procedures and Operations." *Nursing Outlook.* 17:6:36–39. June, 1969. Wayne, D. "School Nursing and Team Teaching." *Nursing Outlook.* 17:7:37. July, 1969. Bonine, G. N. "The Myelogyplastic Child, Hospital and Home Care." *American Journal of Nursing.* 69:3:541–544. March, 1969; direct observation, pediatrician's office, Denver, Colorado, 6/2/69.

65. Rinehart, E. L., *op. cit.,* pp. 192–196.

66. Wall Street Journal. August 4, 1969, p. 1. For general discussion of the delivery of health services in the community, see: National Commission on Community Health Services. *Health Is a Community Affair.* Cambridge, Massachusetts: Harvard University Press. 1966. Also, *Report of the National Advisory Commission on Health Manpower, Volume 1.* Washington, D.C.: U.S. Government Printing Office. 1967. pp. 72-74. Data on the nurse's role are present in many articles and reports, including the previously cited visit to a pediatrician's office in Denver, Colorado and the article by Ford and Silver.

67. Direct observation, pediatrician's office, Denver, Colorado, 6/2/69; Silver, H. K., Ford, L. C., and Stearly, M. S. "A Program to Increase Health Care for Children: The Pediatric Nurse Practitioner Program." *Pediatrics.* 39:5:756–760. May, 1967.

68. Interview, New York-Cornell Hospital, 5/2/69.

69. American Nurses' Association, *supra.,* p. 21.

70. Interview, Tufts University Columbia Point Health Center, Boston, Massachusetts, 2/20/69; interview, Martin Luther King, Jr. Community Center, New York, New York, 7/15/69.

71. National Commission of Community Health Services, *op. cit.* Magraw, R. M. "Inter-disciplinary Teamwork for Medical Care and Health Service." *Annals of Internal Medicine.* 69:4:821–835. October, 1968.

72. Davidson, R. P. and Quick, D. T. "Presentation of a Situation in Which There Has Been Collaboration on Patient Care." *Nurse-Physician Collaboration Toward Improved Patient Care.* New York: American Nurses' Association. 1966. pp. 15–17.

73. For example see: Pinneo, R. "Nursing in a Coronary Care Unit." *American Journal of Nursing.* 65:2:76–79. February, 1965.

74. Lewis, C. E., *op. cit., passim.*

75. Data were extrapolated from: American Nurses' Association. *Facts About Nursing, 1967 Edition.* New York: American Nurses' Association. 1967. p. 15, and *Facts About Nursing, 1968 Edition.* p. 18.

76. Rinehart, E. L., *op. cit.,* pp. 192–196.

77. Peplau, H. "Specialization in Professional Nursing." *Nursing Science.* 3:4:268+. August, 1965.

78. Interview, Kansas City Children's Hospital, Kansas City, Missouri, 5/13/69.

79. Duff, R. S. and Hollingshead, A. B., *op. cit.,* p. 384.

80. *Health Manpower Perspective: 1967, loc. cit.*

81. "The Surgeon General Looks at Nursing." *op. cit.,* p. 67.

82. American Medical Association/American Nurses' Association. *Nurse-Physician Collaboration Toward Improved Patient Care.* New York: American Nurses' Association. 1966. *passim.* Knowles, J. "Medical Care: Its Social and Organizational Aspects." *The New England Journal of Medicine.* 269:8:405–406. August 22, 1963. Pratt, H. "The Doctor's View of the Changing Nurse-Physician Relationship." *Journal of Medical Education.* 40:8:767–771. August, 1965. Selmanoff, E. D. "Strains in the Nurse-Doctor Relationship." *Nursing Clinics of North America.* 3:1:117–127. March, 1968. Hudson, C. "The Changing Medical Climate in America." *Missouri Medicine.* 64:12:965–969. December, 1967. Pellegrino, E. D. "The Physician and the Nurse." *Annals of Internal Medicine.* 64:5:1140–1145. May, 1966. Peplau, H. "Nurse-Doctor Relationships." *Nursing Forum.* 5:1:60+ 1966. Bates, B. "Nurse-Physician Teamwork." *International Nursing Review.* 13:6:53-61. December, 1966.

83. Lewis, C. E., *op. cit.,* p. 63. American Medical Association/American Nurses' Association. *Nurse-Physician Collaboration Toward Improved Patient Care., op. cit.,* pp. 9–10. Statement of Dr. Barbara Bates, member NCSNNE Health Professions Advisory Panel.

84. Lewis, C. E., *op. cit.,* p. 19.

85. U.S. Department of Health, Education, and Welfare, Public Health Service, Division of Nursing. *Current Nursing Research Grants, op. cit.,* pp. 10, 13, 14.

86. Creighton, H. "Operation Gary." *Exploring Progress in Medical-Surgical Nursing Practice.* ANA Regional Clinical Conferences 1965, Vol. 2. New York: American Nurses' Association. 1965. pp. 80–92.

87. Kolthoff, N. J. "The Use of the Laboratory." *Nursing Research.* 16:2:122-124. Spring, 1967.

88. Christman, L. P. and Jelinek, R. C. "Old Patterns Waste Half the Nursing Hours." *op. cit.,* p. 79.

89. Jupiter, Robert. "Patient Transport Service Saves Valuable Nursing Hours." *Hospitals.* 42:6:57. March 16, 1968.

90. Interview, New York-Cornell Hospital, 5/2/69.

91. Lewis, C. E., *op. cit.,* p. 24.

92. American Nurses' Association. "Statement on Graduate Education in Nursing." New York: American Nurses' Association. 1969. p. 2.

93. *Ibid.,* pp. 3–4.

FOUR
FINDINGS AND RECOMMENDATIONS ON
NURSING ROLES AND FUNCTIONS

In recent years, every major health journal in the United States has editorialized on the need to reorganize our health care system. Today, popular magazines have taken up the cause, and the public is reading more than ever about the problems inherent in the way we care for people. Some experienced observers, for example, John Knowles of Massachusetts General Hospital, have predicted that our entire health system will be singled out as a national political issue by the presidential election of 1972.[1] Walter Reuther has already been instrumental in the formation of a political action group called the Committee for National Health Insurance.[2]

This great concern for changing and expanding the present system of health care has vital implications for nursing. In particular, we can trace two related trends that are already apparent. First, there is the development of new congruent relationships between nurses and physicians and between nurses and other health practitioners. This means that the nurse is assuming certain roles that have traditionally belonged to others while divesting herself of functions that are conventionally associated with "the lady in white."

Second, there is the growing emphasis on health maintenance and disease prevention to complement our present system of care for acute, episodic situations. An ounce of prevention may well be worth a pound of cure—and the costs of providing these two services seem to be in the same proportions.

There is little argument that these trends should emerge; rather, the debate centers on specific directions and forms of control. Health costs have grown enormously. By one estimate, the nation spent $63 billion on health services in 1969, with hospital care representing 38 percent of the total.[3] Yet many of these same hospitals are on the narrow edge of financial disaster because their costs exceed their income; a precipitate increase in a single expense area might be more than they could bear.[4]

Today, we are observing more and more activity focused on restructuring roles and locales in relation to health activities. We find physicians and nurses, sometimes together, frequently in independent studies, reexamining their relationships to each other and to the patient. Johnson, Wilcox, and Moidel, for example, see a whole new dimension to the clinical practice of nursing, with the qualified professional assuming major responsibility and accountability for patient care, along with authority to make decisions and control the plan for nursing intervention.[5] Rather than viewing such action as an unwarranted intrusion into the traditional bounds of medicine, the American Medical Association itself has suggested that we might find one solution to our health problems in training 50 to 75 thousand nurses to practice medicine under the supervision of physicians.[6] Although these proposals are broadly related there still remain important semantic and practical differences between them. Only occasionally, as in Idaho, do we find the physician and the nurse actually sitting down together to plan how to manage the practicalities of change in role and responsibility.[7]

The proposals for new emphasis on the distributive practice of health care, i.e., maintenance and prevention, have their antecedents in the public health professions. Indeed, economics and social pressure are combining today to bring this area of practice into more equal partnership with established episodic systems. There is growing evidence that better screening and diagnosis can not only reduce hospital admissions, but also contribute to more effective utilization of facilities and services for those individuals who are admitted.[8]

Related to both these trends is the rapid advance of technology for both episodic and distributive settings. Transplants and multiphasic screening, laser beams and television consultancies, along with developments still on the drawing boards, will continue to elevate the sophistication of treatment and increase the demands on personnel for knowledge and understanding.[9]

To help our staff document current changes in nursing roles and project how these forces might shape the future demands for nurse practitioners, we questioned nurse educators, directors of nursing service, and nurse practitioners in every level and specialty. We also met with individuals, groups, and advisory panels from medicine, health administration, and third party payers. Included, too, were spokesmen for consumer groups, social scientists, economists, and officials of public agencies.

In addition to holding personal interviews, we mailed survey forms to hundreds of individuals and organizations so that we might broaden our base of representation. Searches of the literature, studies of research findings, and on-site visits further supplemented our inquiry into the concerns for nursing practice.

From these various resources and respondents, we have compiled a comprehensive set of requirements for ordering the future development of nursing roles. That is not to say that we can prescribe the roles—for that is beyond the capacity of any individual or commission. **It is possible, however, to suggest mechanisms for ensuring that roles are made, and continue to be remade, relevant for the needs of the times.**

RESEARCH INTO NURSING PRACTICE

This commission assumes as a first principle that excellence in nursing practice results in measurable benefits, in both improved health care and reduced per-patient costs. Thus, we are dismayed that so little research has been done on the actual effects of nursing intervention and care; the profession has few definitive guides for the improvement of practice.

Whether in medicine, engineering, agronomy, or education, scientific research is the key to discovery, to improved practice, and to measurable benefits for society. It is true that each of these disciplines has had to fight, and fight hard, for acceptance of the concept that rigorous research is both necessary and beneficial. For example, when agriculture first appeared among the academic departments of the university, it was ridiculed. The thought that one could have a "science of farming" seemed incredible. Yet, in less than a century, our knowledge of agronomy has given us the capability for growing foodstuffs in incredible abundance.

We can draw a parallel case history from the fantastic strides in medicine. It has been said that until the twentieth century the physician could treat with confidence perhaps only 20 percent of the injuries and diseases that he encountered. For the most part, he could offer the patient only concern, hope, and consolation. As the scientific sphere of medicine has expanded through research, we have been confronted with a dramatically improved picture. A child is spared poliomyelitis by the inquiry of researchers whom he has never seen. An intrauterine transfusion prevents the tragic consequences of Rh incompatibility—a condition that could not even be effectively treated only a decade ago. Psychiatric care rehabilitates an adult whom society would have rejected or confined only a few years earlier. No one questions the fact that we live longer and more productive lives because of medical research and its effects on medical practice.

As Flexner viewed the historic development of American medical education, he observed that " . . . an empirical training of varying excellence, secured through attendance on a preceptor, gave way to the didactic method, which simply communicated a set body of doctrines of very uneven value; . . . to a procedure that seeks, as far as may be, to escape empiricism in order to base the practice of medicine on observed facts of the same order and cogency as pass muster in other fields of pure and applied science."[10] In his seminal report on medical education, he emphasized the need for more understanding of the basic sciences and for inquiry into both basic and applied aspects of science to assure optimum quality of patient care.

The analogy between the phases of medical development and those of nursing is startling. Beginning with the empirical training of nurse attendants in colonial times, through the lectures of Warrington and others who sought to regularize nursing instruction in the 1840's, to the development of a standard curriculum, nursing has tended to recapitulate the experience of medicine.[11] There were essential differences, of course. Nursing always tended to retain some clinical experience even when medicine passed through a period of great reliance on lectures to communicate knowledge to its students. On the other hand, the development of the third, or scientific phase, of nursing education has been restricted. In 1948, Brown could observe, " . . . large numbers of graduate nurses are not professional nurses within this larger meaning. . . . How could they be when one recalls the narrowness and the poverty of the training provided them?"[12]

In the past, nursing has not conducted sufficient research into its own practices. This is a simple statement of fact, not criticism. Nursing has had neither sufficient support for the funding of such inquiries nor enough personnel with the expertise to conduct these rigorous investigations. It is time to change all that.

Lack of research leaves us without a body of facts or a set of probabilities to guide or assess the nursing care of a patient. Of necessity, nursing practice today consists of stereotyped techniques sprinkled liberally with personal idiosyncrasy. What a nurse does, and when, is most frequently determined by pressures in the external setting rather than by any clear knowledge of differential benefit to the patient. Since we have not developed valid means for assessing the effects of varied interventions, it is almost impossible to define optimum nursing care.

The capacity of nursing to gear itself for research into its own techniques is sharply limited. Fewer than 500 American nurses are known to hold doctoral degrees—the generally accepted level for developed research competence.[13]

Within this body of individuals, many are graduates of programs in education, psychology, sociology, and related fields, while less than 20 prepared for the doctorate in physical or biological fields.[14] These figures are reflected in the areas selected for current inquiries into nursing. Of those studies reported in *Nursing Research* during 1969, for example, more investigations have dealt with issues on education and professionalism than with the clinical practice of nursing *per se*.[15]

Where nurses with properly developed research skills have attempted to push back the unknowns on nursing intervention, the results have been most promising. Hoffman and Maibenco have studied postpartum changes in lower organisms and their findings have relevance for the care of maternal patients.[16] Elwood's investigation of physiological responses to breathing exercises for the improved care of patients with chronic lung disease demonstrates the value of even nonsignificant results, in this case showing that certain nursing practices do not really affect outcomes in patients.[17] Pfaudler's investigation of patient response to physical exercises has deep significance for the improved rehabilitation of patients with strokes.[18] Pinneo's studies of coronary care[19] and the work of Resnick and Lewis on ambulatory care[20] further illustrate the impact of greater knowledge on both episodic and distributive nursing interventions.

These few examples underscore the need for major thrusts in nursing research. This commission believes it is essential for the future of health care in the United States to begin a systematic evaluation of the impact of nursing care. We advocate the development of objective criteria such as measurable improvement in patient condition, evidence of early discharge or return to employment, reduced incidence of readmission to care facilities, and lowered rates of communicable disease. We do not suggest for a moment that nursing is wholly responsible for these or any other facet in the total health care picture. We do believe, however, that nursing represents an important independent variable. As such, we must learn how we can utilize our nurses more effectively, more efficiently, and more economically.

In these concerns about research, nursing is not unique. Each profession has had to develop its own commitment in this area. And each profession has experienced the frustrations of insufficient personnel, inadequate funds, and skepticism about the values of theory and inquiry.

Once the general public begins to reap the fruits of such study, however, it can be counted on to provide continuing support for further inquiry. This means, of course, that public and private agencies plus state and federal governments must invest initial seed money to launch the initial studies that are sorely needed in nursing. In the last fiscal year, for example, less than $4,000,000 was allocated to investigations in nursing, including traineeships for advanced research students. In contrast, more than $40 million was provided for medical research. We must begin to build from this point toward expanded investigations into the practice and effects of nursing care. We recommend that:

> 1. *The federal Division of Nursing, the National Center for Health Services Research and Development, other governmental agencies, and private foundations appropriate grant funds and/or research contracts to investigate the impact of nursing practice on the quality, effectiveness, and economy of health care.*

Because there is so much to be done within such limited resources at the outset, nursing should avoid duplication of effort and, at the same time, ensure broad dissemination of results. For these reasons, we would encourage the immediate establishment of a national clearinghouse for nursing research to collect, catalogue, and distribute information on investigations completed or in progress. We recommend that:

> 2. *Federal funds be supplied through the ERIC* program, or through the Division of Nursing, as well as private and state funds, to the American Nurses' Foundation so that it might become a national clearinghouse for the collection and dissemination of information about research and innovations in nursing.*

There is a crucial need for basic research in nursing practice; in addition, support should be made available for applied research and demonstration projects that can serve as model applications of research findings. In our society, a cultural lag tends to intervene between discovery and application. In the case of nursing, with its profound influence on the delivery of optimum health care, we must be concerned that research findings are translated with speed into application and changed practice. In order to encourage innovation in nursing practice, we recommend that:

> 3. *The Division of Nursing, the National Center for Health Services Research and Development, and state and private funds allocate increased monies for applied research and demonstration grants that would examine new methods, procedures, settings, and personnel relationships for improved nursing practice. We further recommend that the following guidelines be used in expending funds:*
>
> a. *Innovation and demonstration projects in patient care should be based on preceding research;*
>
> b. *Innovations should be conceived and focused to improve methods of meeting patient needs, rather than designed primarily to answer professional problems;*
>
> c. *All grants and contracts for applied research and demonstrations should include an allocation for the evaluation of results;*
>
> d. *All innovations and demonstrations should be weighed against alternative courses of action that might produce similar results. Both quality of care and comparative costs should be considered.*

*Educational Research Information Center

In addition to determining how basic research findings can apply to nursing practice, the use of demonstration and applied research may also lead to the evaluation of nursing in terms of the objective criteria we outlined above. For example, researchers may find that a therapeutic measure used under controlled conditions can be assessed in such terms as improved patient condition, evidence of early discharge, and reduced incidence of readmission. Moreover, such procedures, examined within the complete research design, can contribute to information about the economics of alternative courses of nursing practice. The substitution of personnel, the costs of training or supervision, and other current intangibles may be analyzed more objectively once we have baseline data for optimum nursing care.

This commission emphasizes its belief that basic and applied research is essential to adequate knowledge about nursing practice. Further, we hold that once initial discoveries and applications prove their worth, continuing support will be found. Nursing itself must assume major responsibility to ensure that individuals undertake research and to encourage other individuals and agencies to evaluate the results. There is every reason to believe that nursing will find as much value inherent in its research as other professions. Indeed, research and applied learning have forged the professionalism of these other groups. The health care system, and the individual user of that system, stand to be the chief beneficiaries of greater knowledge and predictability in nursing practice.

ROLE ARTICULATION IN HEALTH PRACTICE

To provide the number of qualified nurses needed to cope with the problems of health care delivery in the United States, we must clarify nursing roles and reorganize the career patterns for nursing practice. In essence, nursing must be allowed—and required—to practice at its very highest capability.

It is an old saying that nursing's role is defined by what needs to be done; unfortunately, it is often true. On the job, nurses are frequently called on to perform challenging tasks for which they are not formally prepared, as well as burdensome duties that do not utilize their full knowledge and skills. In an eight-hour period, for example, an individual might function as a pharmacist, an administrator, a housekeeper—and a sometime nurse. In our current situation, faced with a nursing manpower shortage, we need to examine these patterns critically. As the largest of the health professions, and as one of our most precious resources, nursing must function at its best if we are to meet the demand for episodic and distributive care.

In this context, it is not surprising that there are problems and conflicts in spelling out congruent roles between nurses and the other health professionals.

Changing one's patterns of behavior is a threatening, sometimes painful, process and it is often difficult for individuals to accept new roles.[21] Further, when conflict over demarcation of roles breaks out, there can be action and reaction that escalate to the point of organizational warfare.[22] Finally, there is the latent problem that exists when any group unilaterally defines roles for interacting groups.[23]

Role theory, by definition, requires the presence of role congruency. That is, one cannot have the parent role without a role for the child, a leader role without a follower role, or a peer role without an equal's role. Such congruent roles must be arrived at by interaction between the principals, if there is to be cooperation, understanding, and effective role accomplishment.

There is a sterling example of the lack of communication between the health professions in terms of role development: the proposal to solve the health problems of the country, in part, by having nurses practice medicine under the supervision of a physician. According to the article in which this was suggested, the American Medical Association had cleared the proposal with officials of the American Hospital Association, but apparently had not spoken to nurses, at least through their professional organization, the American Nurses' Association.[24]

To a degree, the proposal itself is consistent with both the clinical capabilities demonstrated by an increasing number of nurses and the desires of even more nurses to see their professional skills match the challenge of their job responsibilities. The key to action, however, lies in the discussion and development of the role of the nurse in *mutual cooperation* with other health care professions. As one nursing leader has stated flatly, "We don't want to be physicians' assistants."[25] This reaction is understandable and predictable when viewed from a basic understanding of human behavior. Decisions, to be binding, must be made in a spirit of mutual confidence.

This commission recognizes that each profession has the right and responsibility to assess its own roles, but the critical need for joint action demands that congruent roles be articulated and planned among the professions. Within the past few years, a number of promising avenues for role change in nursing and medicine have been developed. Some have come to a dead end because of the suspicion, fear of domination, and simple lack of understanding that have characterized past relationships. Even now, however, there are some encouraging signs.

A series of joint conferences on nurse-physician relationships has been sponsored by the American Nurses' Association and the American Medical Association.[26] The success of these discussions and the recognition of·the contributions of coworkers in medicine and nursing led to the recent recommendation that further conferences be held at the state level.[27]

Relatedly, a number of meetings have occurred in the past several years where physicians and nurses met to discuss technical matters related to state health practice acts. When new treatments or procedures arise, where roles change, or where legal liability is clouded, interprofessional conferences have been successful in resolving the role relationships between the physician and the nurse.[28] While these joint statements and policies are limited in scope, they are an indication that wider areas of role interaction are possible.

There is little doubt that sufficient groundwork has been laid. When our staff surveyed a sample of the professional societies and organizational representatives for their reactions to various aspects of relationship, we asked whether further discussions on congruent roles between nurses and physicians would be desirable. The results were overwhelmingly favorable; 85 percent of the state medical societies, 96 percent of the state nurse associations, and 93 percent of the boards of nurse examiners expressed their support for such meetings. Moreover, approximately 90 percent of the same respondents felt that through positive role redefinition nurses could meet special needs of population groups and provide care in areas where it is not adequate now.

Given the success of many of these preliminary steps, and the need for wider areas of agreement on congruent roles to enhance health care, this commission recommends that:

> 4. *A national joint practice commission be established between medicine and nursing to discuss and make recommendations concerning the congruent roles of the physician and the nurse in providing quality health care, with particular attention to the rise of the nurse master clinician; the introduction of the physician's assistant; the increased activity of other professions in areas long assumed to be the concern solely of the physician and/or the nurse.*

Because of the need to examine role relationships in terms of the various state health practice acts, it is essential that discussions be undertaken at this level. The existence of joint commissions within each state, in addition to the national body, would provide expanded opportunity for the exchange and cross-fertilization of ideas. Therefore, we recommend that:

> 5. *Counterpart joint practice commissions be established in each state between medicine and nursing to consider the congruent roles of physicians and nurses, and to recommend to state legislatures and to the national joint practice commission such changes or alterations in basic health practice acts, licensure, and other regulations as they deem necessary to ensure the provision of quality health care.*

Further, the commission recognizes that other individual and organizational roles are involved in the clarification of health care activities. We have suggested that medicine and nursing begin these joint practice discussions because they have current concerns that must be resolved, as well as the background of preliminary activities. As agreements and understandings emerge, these two groups should seek to involve other key members of the health professions. The objective, of course, is to develop more extensive consensus on how to provide and apportion roles for optimum health care. We recommend that:

> 6. *As early as progress in these joint discussions indicates, the national and state joint practice commissions should invite health management executives, other professions and allied health personnel, as well as the rising number of groups involved in health maintenance, disease prevention, and patient care to join in planning for optimum working relationships and concerted role performance that will assure the best delivery of quality health care.*

There is every assurance that medicine and nursing can make salutary progress through discussion and joint planning. It is our sincere hope that their agreement may also serve as an encouragement to the enlarged interdisciplinary groups in the effort to resolve the vexing problems of role confusion and organizational boundaries.

ORGANIZATION OF NURSING ROLES

Even before the role definitions that will grow out of the joint practice commissions, the profession must cope with the problems of providing a sufficient number of nurses for a diversified health care delivery system while at the same time making a career in nursing practice more intrinsically rewarding.

It seems obvious that the simplest solution to any shortage of nurses in practice would be to bring back large numbers of the 286,000 licensed inactive individuals. This "simple solution" is difficult to translate into reality, however. In comparison with all female baccalaureate graduates, for example, nurses demonstrate a lower percentage of active career participation at almost all points across a time line.[29]

It would appear also that the inherent rewards of the profession, at least with regard to actual nursing practice, are simply not sufficient to induce nurses to remain in their careers. In part, this situation stems from the economics of nursing salaries. A recent report by the American Hospital Association showed that 75 percent of the community hospitals pay less than $7,500 a year for practicing nurses.[30] This matter is of such concern that it is treated at length in Chapter Six, yet this is not the sole problem in any consideration of career practice.

There is abundant testimony that the direct care of patients is the most satisfying single aspect of their profession for a majority of nurses. Nevertheless, the nurse in practice is very apt to find that 50 to 75 percent of her time is spent in non-nursing functions.[31] The available opportunities for direct patient care are limited by the necessities for passing medications, maintaining records, and handling clerical and supervisory activities.[32] Indeed, promotion tends to take the nurse further away from direct clinical practice to a managerial function of overseeing care provided by others, often nonprofessionals.[33]

In response to our survey, nurses and physicians, and to a lesser extent health administrators, were in overwhelming agreement that the nursing role has absorbed far too many administrative and other non-nursing functions. Correspondingly, our on-site visits gave us the opportunity to talk to individuals from many fields about their observations of nursing satisfaction. Their responses tend to confirm the general analyses of motivation suggested by Herzberg[34] and Myers[35] from their studies in industrial psychology. Thus, nurses would probably be most satisfied when they have the opportunity to engage in practice, and to perform these tasks fully and well; have responsibility for what they do; and gain recognition for accomplishment. The more qualified the nurse, the more she desires independence and latitude of judgment. Optimum conditions should exist when nurses are able to concentrate on care activities and can rely on others to carry out related but non-nursing functions.

All this suggests that career patterns must be developed to keep nurses in practice. This means that new forms of recognition and compensation are needed, and, in view of the changing nature of health care delivery, companion careers must be arranged for emerging areas in our health system.

The hospital nurse, important as she is to the care of the acutely ill, represents only one segment of a full health service plan. The nurse in a neighborhood clinic, occupied with education of parents and examinations of children, represents a different dimension of our health resources. The maintenance of health and the prevention of disease are our best guarantees that the rising costs and overcrowding of our acute care facilities can be controlled. The education of nurses must allow for this differentiation, and career attractiveness must be developed for both kinds of nursing practice.

Our entire health delivery system is groping for a way to help people and treat problems before events reach the catastrophic proportions that require in-patient institutional care. It is essential that we develop nurses for both kinds of practice and that we plan for the requirements of these differing role situations. We recommend that:

> 7. *Two essentially related but differing career patterns be developed for nursing practice:*
> a. *One career pattern, episodic, would emphasize the nursing practice that is*

essentially curative and restorative, generally acute or chronic in nature, and most frequently provided in the setting of the hospital or in-patient facility;

   b. The second career pattern, distributive, would emphasize the nursing practice that is essentially designed for health maintenance and disease prevention. This is generally continuous in nature, seldom acute, and increasingly will take place in community or emergent institutional settings.

This two-fold emphasis in nursing practice stems from the pragmatic appraisal of the need to provide better lifelong health care and preventive measures that can reduce the incidence of catastrophic illness or disease. As Millis has noted, "Health care to many means medical cure. Nurses are educated to care. Cure is an event, by nature and episode. Care is a process, not an event, and is lifelong. Yet major efforts and funds are given to cure which represents less than 25 percent of service."[36] Today, almost two out of three nurses are engaged in hospital settings. The remainder are spread thinly in all other areas of practice. It is essential that we readjust our perspectives toward the locus of nursing care at the same time that we make careers more satisfying regardless of location. For this reason, we recommend that:

   8. Both nursing career patterns should be so organized that recognition, reward, and increased responsibility for practice are based on increasing depth of knowledge and demonstrated competence to perform in complex clinical situations.

It is important to emphasize the continuance of nursing practice, and to attach rewards to demonstrated competence. At the same time, it is essential that the profession develop an enhanced career perspective that recognizes levels of capability and provides for both monetary and other rewards as a result of performance. This commission recommends that:

   9. Within each functional specialty, episodic or distributive, a career plan should be developed by which beginning nurse graduates would start at an entry level (staff nurse) then move to increased levels of competence (clinical nurse). In this position, the nurse might function as a nursing team leader in clinical practice. With proper experience and advanced study, an individual could be recognized as a master clinician capable of organizing and providing complex care using initiative and individual judgment.

In such a career plan, terms like generalist and specialist are determined by the individual situation. For example, the master clinician in cardiovascular care (episodic) might be termed a specialist, while the master clinician in family health care (distributive) might better be viewed as a highly capable generalist.

We have long had the pattern of the public health nurse, with her specialty superimposed on her preparation in hospital nursing. In the growing complexity of health care, and in the widening demands for nursing practice, it seems less possible than ever before to prepare every nursing student to function in all situations. On the other hand, we feel too narrow a specialization would not be in the best interests of either the nurse or the public. Thus, it appears that these two general fields, episodic and distributive care, provide a sufficient range of activities, plus ample opportunity for cross-relationships. This structure, we feel, can avoid too narrow an approach while affording reasonable contexts for concentration.

During our on-site visits, we have also had an opportunity to examine the institutional beginnings of structured levels in nursing competence. At Case Western Reserve, for example, a series of gradations based on demonstrated competence has been put into use. The results indicate that nurses do find a positive inducement in reward and recognition for outstanding practice.[37] At Massachusetts General Hospital, a slightly different arrangement of recognition through clinical levels has had promising results.[38]

We must underscore the fact that redirection of nursing time and effort toward actual practice must be accompanied by a divestment of the non-nursing functions that currently occupy so much time. The potential of industrial engineering surveys, together with the advancements of modern technology, should permit us to find ways to accomplish these tasks safely and efficiently by personnel other than nurses. We recommend that:

> 10. *All clerical, technical, and routine supportive functions which are not therapeutic be performed by non-nursing personnel. These would include the provision of supplies, maintenance of records, supervision of housekeeping services, and related activities.*

A current study under the auspices of the Vanderbilt University School of Nursing indicates that it is possible to make careful discriminations between nursing and non-nursing (or stewardess) functions. This kind of approach will allow professional personnel to provide their unique services while routine maintenance functions are carried out by others.[39]

Relatedly, we need to reexamine our organizational structures and practices to ensure that inertia and tradition do not perpetuate the use of professional personnel for non-nursing tasks. This commission recommends that:

> 11. *Continuous study be given to the provision of ward clerks, unit managers, self-contained departments, automated services, and other organizational departures that can release nurses from non-nursing functions while maintaining nursing control over the delivery of nursing care.*

Finally, we discovered, in both our examination of the literature and our site visits, that innovative changes in one organization had not been adopted by others. In part, this problem stemmed from the fact that individuals might experiment with change, but they would make no provision for evaluating results or communicating the new practice. Frequently when the individual leaves, the innovation passes—sometimes to be rediscovered by someone else, sometimes to be forgotten. In order to determine the actual worth of these changes, and to replace anecdotal evidence with something more tangible, we recommend that:

> 12. *Each change in handling and procedure be accompanied with educational programs and followed by evaluative procedures to ensure that organizational changes are accompanied by actual increases in nursing time for health delivery and by qualitative improvements in care.*

Through earnest efforts to have nurses practice nursing, and simultaneously ensure that their non-nursing work is taken up by others, we have the potential to produce not only more care, but also more satisfaction for those who enter this profession because it offers the possibility of providing direct, individual care for those in need of it. If we could recover only a portion of the time now spent by nurses in non-nursing duties, if we could reactivate only a percentage of the available nurses through the promise of enhanced opportunities for practice, then manpower shortages might be relieved. Even more important, the standards and quality of care should improve simply through greater emphasis on and recognition of skilled nursing practice.

LEADERSHIP FOR NURSING PRACTICE

Closely related to the effort to develop a continuing career prospective for nurse practitioners is the need to redirect the leadership of nursing roles. Traditionally, nursing service administration has lacked a clear voice in the policy- and decision-making bodies of the health organizations. To ensure that the increased clinical competence in nursing is utilized most effectively, we urge that nursing leadership be included in deliberations concerning health care in both institutional and community settings.[40]

The elevation of nursing service to a level of full partnership with medicine and health management is overt organizational recognition of the importance of nursing care in the total configuration of patient needs. It is an acknowledgment that planning, coordinating, and conduct of nursing care is a prime concern of the health care facility.

To invest nursing with this authority requires the assumption of great responsibility on the part of the profession. Nursing must accept the full burden of conducting its own affairs and working on joint problems as well. However, such a plan demands that the administration of nursing practice, both episodic and distributive, reside with clinical directors who are qualified to plan, organize, and direct nursing care.

One example of such a plan is illustrated in the organization of the Evanston Hospital.[41] This institution has established an independent Patient Care Council that reports to the board of directors. The group includes the chiefs of medicine, surgery, obstetrics-gynecology, nursing, and health administration. The policies determined by this council are arrived at jointly and apply to all aspects of patient care. This same approach operates at the unit level with service triads of physicians, nurses, and administrators.

On the basis of this and several other experimental organizations, as well as the judgment of our advisory panels, this commission recommends that:

> 13. *Institutional policy-making and administrative bodies in health care facilities (both episodic and distributive) should be so organized that the clinical director of nursing service has a voice in planning and decisions that affect the provision of health care, and that medicine, nursing, and health administration join together for mutual discussion of their common concerns in optimizing care delivery.*

Any number of approaches can be used to help facilitate joint planning and decision making. At some locations, for example, there is concerted effort to include all representatives in patient conferences and care planning meetings. In other settings medical and nursing students have joined with professional practitioners for combined patient rounds and visitation. Similarly, joint committees have been formed to develop institutional procedures and directives. Each of these measures is elemental recognition of the contributions and special capabilities of the individuals and groups involved. From the standpoint of resultant care, Wilbur has remarked that such team concepts will ". . . bring services to patients. Together we will accomplish what neither of us [nurses and doctors] can accomplish alone. This requires much collaboration."[42]

There can be no doubt that nursing practice needs leadership in the form of strengthened clinical directors, i.e., persons responsible for managing nursing practice and for working cooperatively with other professions in joint planning of care. At the same time, it is essential that a *rapprochement* be established between the twin specialties of nursing service and nursing education. In the historical span of the profession, education and service were once combined in the diploma school of nursing. When the education process was transferred to separate institutions, partly in reaction to the demands on student time by nursing service, a split occurred that has not yet healed completely. In a growing number of institutions, improved communication and cooperation have taken place through individual efforts and through organizational action. In particular, a number of collegiate institutions with affiliated health centers have restored the concept of appointing one head for both education and service. This approach helps to ensure that planning does involve mutual considerations of clinical service and teaching. Such a reestablishment of relations is essential not only to improve communication but also to ensure the widespread dissemination of advances in practice, theory, and research. As such, it is incumbent upon the leaders of nursing practice, as well as leaders in nursing education, to strive for mutual planning and policy making. Nursing students need to have a consistent professional orientation to their clinical experience, and this requires consistent two-way communication between nurse educators and practitioners. We recommend that:

> 14. *Nursing leadership work actively to bring education and service together in joint planning and decision making, and that where practicable*
> a. *Nurse practitioners and clinical directors of nursing service receive significant appointments to (or relevant association with) institutions for nursing education, and*
> b. *Nursing faculty in institutions for nursing education be given responsibility for providing or organizing significant elements of nursing care.*

Out of this approach can come the development of the professional nurse career that is not wholly bifurcated between practice and teaching. The contribution of these two elements to improved nursing practice is too great to continue in the present, separated status.

TECHNOLOGY AND CHANGING SYSTEMS

Out of the advances in health science, and particularly the applications of increased technology to the delivery of therapy, have come a myriad of new opportunities—and new difficulties. The use of electronic monitors in intensive care units, for instance, has aided dramatically in the effective care of the patient. Simultaneously, these instruments have freed the attending nurse from performing routine and repetitive measurements, allowing her to concentrate on patient management.[43] This advance, however, as emphasized strongly by Crosby, does not eliminate the need for a very special nurse who can interpret and swiftly initiate appropriate responses at the computer's signal.[44] In other words, while advanced technology eliminates certain routines and even some of the lower skill operations, it introduces the need for persons with new knowledge and the capacity to assume responsibility for individual action.

So pervasive is the effect of technology, accompanied by the dramatic advances in epidemiology, transplantation, and screening, that our surveys of the health professional were in near-unanimous agreement that the future practice of nursing will be substantially different from the present. There was general agreement that in some cases the nurse would have to learn to operate new equipment; there was also acceptance of the fact that nurses would need to adjust to new opportunities for patient care based on the elimination of current procedures as well as the assumption of new activities. Recognizing the profound impacts that these changes will have on the roles and functions of nurses, this commission urges nursing to continue to explore the application of new discoveries to enhance health care. Specifically, we recommend that:

15. *Nurses seek to use technology in their activities for two primary purposes:*

a. *To eliminate as much routine as possible, allowing them to achieve maximum personal contact with their charges;*

b. *To enlarge the monitoring and feedback systems that can supply information on individual conditions and reactions, thus facilitating further nursing intervention.*

Along with the advances in technology, we must remain aware of the human aspects of modern patient care. Almost every individual facing health problems (particularly those concerned with episodic treatment) experiences physical and emotional stress. Feelings of loneliness and alienation are present, at least in latent form, even under the best of conditions. The seeming impersonality of advanced techniques of therapy can affect the perception of the individual, and even the progress of his reaction to treatment.[45]

In light of these circumstances, some one professional is required to serve as an overall coordinator and interpreter of the plan for care. This means that someone must relate directly and humanly with the patient, while also assuming responsibility for the cooperative activities carried out by the host of professionals who are involved in today's program of total treatment. It is in both the tradition and the particular capabilities of nursing to serve as this organizational link—to relate to both patient and professional and to translate from one to the other. To assure the continued humane concern for the individual, and to provide for the coordination of professional intervention, this commission recommends that:

16. *Clinical nurses, in both episodic and distributive settings, assume responsibility for:*

a. *Seeing that every nursing action evidences an interest and concern for the individual;*

b. *Facilitating the efforts of other health care personnel in providing for the needs of an individual.*

Obviously, such a proposal anticipates that the nurse will play the role of intermediary in future health care. That is, in the development of a regimen of treatment, the nurse will occupy a crucial position between the patient and most other health professionals. She will ensure that communications between them are understood and carried out. She will also relate to the individual patient as the central person for aid and interpretation. Of necessity, she will assume a crucial role in applying technology and therapy to individual treatment. It is essential that the patient's personal feelings be taken into account and individual worth be recognized. Moreover, the very success of advanced technology and therapeutic intervention will depend on the variations and adjustments that are made in relation to the individual patient. The nurse is in a unique position to observe and determine these differences, and it is on the nurse that excellence in individualized treatment will depend.

In view of the simultaneous need for enlarging the dimensions of nursing and health care, and for caring for far greater numbers of individuals in both episodic and distributive settings, we recommend that:

> 17. *Nursing educators and practitioners place continuing emphasis on the role of the nurse:*
>
> a. *As a central figure in the provision of psychosocial as well as physical care for the patient and his family;*
>
> b. *As a representative of the individual care recipient and his interests in inter- or multidisciplinary approaches to the delivery of health care.*

Ultimately, the entire health care delivery system of the country must be judged by its capacity to deal with the requirements of thousands of individuals and their families. Mass inoculations, large efforts at screening, vast educational programs all have merit and relevance. However, it is in the intimacy and immediacy of individual problems that we shall maintain—or lose—the viability of our system. On the nurse rests a major portion of the ultimate responsibility for seeing that health care is dispensed with dignity and concern.

FOOTNOTES

1. Knowles, J. "The Physician in the Decade Ahead." *Hospitals.* 44:1:58. January 1, 1970.
2. "Committee for National Health Insurance Tells What It Wants in Federal Plan." *Modern Hospital.* 114:1:97–102. January 1, 1970.
3. Faltermeyer, E. K. "Better Care at Less Cost Without Miracles." *Fortune.* 81:1:81. January, 1970. Percentage extrapolated from graph.
4. American Hospital Association. *Annual Reports–1969.* Chicago: American Hospital Association. 1969. p. 86.

5. Johnson, D. E., Wilcox, J. A., and Moidel, H. C. "The Clinical Specialist as a Practitioner." *American Journal of Nursing.* 67:11:2298-2303. November, 1967.

6. Rowan, C. "AMA to Push Radical Plan to Spread Health Care." *Democrat and Chronicle.* Rochester, New York. December 28, 1969. p. 2E.

7. Raphael, Sister Mary. "The Development and Activities of a Joint Physician-Nurse Liaison Committee." *Report of the AMA Conference Sponsored by the AMA Committee on Nursing.* American Medical Association. 1967.

8. Knowles, J., *op. cit.,* p. 60.

9. *Technology and Manpower in the Health Service Industry 1965-75.* U.S. Department of Labor, Manpower Administration. May, 1967. pp. 35-60.

10. Flexner, A. *Medical Education in the United States and Canada.* Boston: D. B. Updike, The Merrymount Press. 1960. p. 20.

11. Bullough, V. L. and Bullough, B. *The Emergence of Modern Nursing, Second Edition.* New York: The Macmillan Company. 1969. pp. 120-147.

12. Brown, E. L. *Nursing for the Future.* New York: Russell Sage Foundation. 1948. p. 75.

13. American Nurses' Foundation. "Directory of Nurses with Earned Doctoral Degrees." *Nursing Research.* 18:5:465-480. September-October, 1969.

14. *Ibid.*

15. *Nursing Research.* 18:1. January-February, 1969. 18:2. March-April, 1969. 18:3. May-June, 1969. 18:4. July-August, 1969. 18:5. September-October, 1969. 18:6. November-December, 1969.

16. Hoffman, Joan C. "Timing of Pituitary LH Release Responsible for Postpartum and 'Progesterone Withdrawal' Ovulation in the Rat." University of Illinois. 1965. Unpublished doctoral dissertation. See also: *Dissertation Abstracts-1967.* 27B:2852. Maibenco, Helen C. "Connective Tissue Changes in Postpartum Uterine Involution in the Albino Rat." *Anatomical Record.* 136:59-70. 1960.

17. Elwood, Evelyn. "Study of Selected Physiological Responses to Breathing Exercise Practice in Patients with Chronic Obstructive Pulmonary Disease." New York University. 1967. Unpublished doctoral dissertation. See also: *Dissertation Abstracts-1968.* 28A:3883.

18. "Self-Instruction for Stroke Victims." Bulletin of the Clearinghouse on Self-Instructional Materials for Health Care Facilities. 3:4. April, 1969. For more complete information see: Final Report. PHS Grant No. NU 00250 "Self-Instruction for Stroke Patients."

19. Pinneo, R. "Nursing in a Coronary Care Unit." *American Journal of Nursing.* 65:2:76-79. February, 1965.

20. Lewis, C. E. and Resnik, B. A. "Nurse Clinics and Progressive Ambulatory Patient Care." *The New England Journal of Medicine.* 277:23:1237-1241. December 7, 1967.

21. The problem of change in role on the security of nurses in administrative positions was reported at many of the sites visited in this study. The general nature of the problem in changing roles is knowledgeably discussed in Schlotfeldt, R. and MacPhail, J. "An Experiment in Nursing: Introducing Planned Change." *American Journal of Nursing.* 69:6:1247-1251. June, 1969.

22. "American Society of Medical Technologists Files Law Suit Against American Society of Clinical Pathologists." *American Society of Medical Technologists News.* 4:11:1. June, 1969.

23. Rowan, C., *op. cit.*

24. *Ibid.*

25. Lambertsen, E. C. "Can We Afford Nursing Care?" Address to the 1968 Convention of the American Nurses' Association. Dallas, Texas. May 15, 1968.

26. *Medical and Nursing Practice in a Changing World.* First National Conference for Professional Nurses and Physicians. 1964. *Nurse-Physician Collaboration Toward Improved Patient Care.* Second National Conference for Professional Nurses and Physicians. 1966. *The Sick Person Needs.* Third National Conference for Professional Nurses and Physicians. 1967. Chicago and New York: American Medical Association/American Nurses' Association. *Report of the AMA Committee on Nursing Sponsored Conference.* Chicago: American Medical Association. 1967.
27. *The Sick Person Needs., op. cit.,* p. 43.
28. "Summary Report of SNA Activities Related to Professional Aspects of Nursing Practice During 1968." New York: American Nurses' Association. 1968.
29. *Health Manpower Perspective: 1967.* Public Health Service Publication No. 1667. Washington, D.C.: U.S. Government Printing Office. 1967. p. 38.
30. American Hospital Association., *op. cit.,* p. 86.
31. Christman, L. and Jelinek, R. C. "Old Patterns Waste Half the Nursing Hours." *Modern Hospital.* 108:1:79. January, 1967.
32. Jacobs, S. E. "Older Patients Get More Care." *Hospitals.* 43:24:71. December 16, 1969.
33. Christman, L. "What the Future Holds for Nursing." Paper presented at a meeting of the California Regional Medical Programs' Conference for Allied Health Professions. April 23, 1969. Pacific Grove, California. Author's Manuscript. pp. 1–3.
34. Herzberg, I., Mausner, B., and Snyderman, B. *The Motivation to Work, Second Edition.* New York: John Wiley & Sons. 1959.
35. Myers, M. S. "Who Are Your Motivated Workers?" *Harvard Business Review.* 42:2:73. January–February, 1964.
36. "National League for Nursing Convention: Detroit May 19–23." *Nursing Outlook.* 17:6:49. June, 1969.
37. Schlotfeldt, R. and MacPhail, J. "Experiment in Nursing: Implementing Planned Change." *American Journal of Nursing.* 69:7:1475–80. July, 1969.
38. Interview, Massachusetts General Hospital, 2/18/69.
39. Interviews, Vanderbilt University Hospital and School of Nursing, 11/14/69. For additional details see: Christman, L. "Would a Stewardess Help?" *Saturday Review.* February 4, 1967. pp. 65–67.
40. Hauer, R. M. "Perspective on Directing Hospital Nursing Service." *American Journal of Nursing.* 69:12:2629. December, 1969. Lambertsen, E. C. "Reorganize Nursing to Re-emphasize Care." *Modern Hospital.* 108:1:68–71+. January, 1967.
41. Interview, Evanston Hospital, Evanston, Illinois, 6/5/69.
42. "National League for Nursing Convention: Detroit May 19–23." *op. cit.,* p. 48.
43. Peplau, H. E. "Automation: Will It Change Nurses, Nursing or Both?" *Technical Innovations in Health Care: Nursing Implications.* American Nurses' Association Clinical Sessions Series No. 5. New York: American Nurses' Association. 1962. pp. 37–48.
44. Crosby, E. L. "Hospitals as the Center of the Health Care Universe." *Hospitals.* 44:1:54. January 1, 1970.
45. Duff, R. S. and Hollingshead, A. B. *Sickness and Society.* New York: Harper & Row. 1968. pp. 151–213, 291–362 and *passim.*

FIVE

FINDINGS AND RECOMMENDATIONS ON NURSING EDUCATION

One of the most vital—and controversial—areas in nursing today is the professional programs for preparation and specialization. Nursing education has been subjected to periodic examination from the days of the Bellevue Hospital School in 1873; from the time of the Goldmark[1] study in 1923, there have been intensive efforts to restructure the institutions and curricula that serve nursing education.

Over the years, some studies, like that of Brown,[2] have examined the entire spectrum of educational programs; others, like those of Montag[3] and Bridgman[4] have concentrated on specific types of institutions. At the state or regional level, we have identified more than 40 studies within the last five years. All these efforts have been characterized by recommendations for change. Differences, as they exist in findings and recommendations, revolve about the issue of whether change can be gradual or not. Some investigators suggest that alterations in present institutions and programs could solve the problems of nursing education; others see the best hope in a radical restructuring of the entire system.

During the time when proposals were being drafted for the formation of this national study of nursing, the issues in nursing education were highlighted by the publication of the American Nurses' Association 1965 position paper and the reactions to that document. The ANA proposed that all preparatory nursing programs be located within institutions of higher education. Some nurses, and even more physicians and administrators, opposed any change in the hospital schools that currently graduate two out of three American nurses.

Proponents of the position paper argued for the academic advantages of regular educational institutions; opponents stressed the merits of the single-purpose program. The controversy escalated. Charges and countercharges abounded. Meanwhile, prospective nursing students, their parents, and the general public were left in confusion.

Obviously, the position paper sparked the venting of long-held feelings by spokesmen for both sides. Rather than acting as a catharsis, however, the controversy heightened animosity and froze organizational attitudes. All this occurred at the time when the new commission was preparing to examine the underlying causes and suggest independent solutions. Thus, one of the first tasks of the study staff was to determine basic facts about nursing education and separate these from feelings, and even from fantasy. Only then could we begin to construct a coherent and useful picture of the needs, resources, and objectives of nursing education.

Our first step was to ask the deans, heads, or directors of each existing nursing program what their greatest problems were and what specific changes would be most helpful to them. Similar inquiries were addressed to the heads of each harboring institution, i.e., hospital administrators and college or university presidents. In addition, the staff sent inquiries to institutions that had recently closed their nursing programs, asking for the reasons and problems that led to their decision. Finally, questionnaires were directed to educational institutions that might have been expected to offer preparatory programs in nursing but did not. We wanted to find out why. From all these returns, we developed our analysis of the problems of institutions for nursing education.

However, institutions are not the sole source of information. Questionnaires were prepared for random samplings of faculty and students to explore their perception of the educational system and the particular strengths and weaknesses of their own preparation. These questionnaires were distributed by means of a random, stratified sample so that institutional and sectional differences could be adequately expressed.

From these replies, and from a close search of the literature, the staff developed preliminary findings. These results were distributed to a large number of organizations, including state nurses' associations, state leagues of nursing, state boards of nursing, state medical societies, state hospital associations, state health departments, representatives of consumers and third-party payers, plus a host of individuals. Their comments provided us with an assessment of consensus as well as a means for determining local and regional variations.

The information obtained on the survey forms and questionnaires was subjected to comparison testing by means of site visits, literature searches, consultation with specialists, and the commentary of our permanent advisory panels.

The results of these analyses may be grouped under eight areas of findings
and recommendations. In total, they embody a national plan for the reorganization
and qualitative improvement of nursing education in the United States, together
with specific indications for implementation and direction.

INSTITUTIONAL PATTERNS FOR NURSING EDUCATION

From the beginnings of nursing education in the United States, the hospital has
been the locus of institutional programs. While there were a small number of collegiate programs in nursing as early as the first decades of the twentieth century,
the overwhelming majority of preparatory sequences were, and are, in the hospital
locale. Most of our current practitioners have received their initial training in these
institutions.

As early as 1923, however, Goldmark noted, ". . . the average hospital training
school is not organized on such a basis as to conform to the standards accepted in
other educational fields . . . instruction in such schools is frequently casual and un-
correlated."[5] Brown, in contrast, described a number of "Distinguished Hospital
Schools" in her report of 1948, and commented on their educational quality; yet
she warned that even these outstanding schools needed the resources of collegiate
instruction to maintain their excellence.[6]

In the years between and following these investigations, criticism and acco-
lades for the institutional patterns of nursing education appeared. Admirers of the
hospital-based system spoke of the emphasis on clinical excellence and the importance of the care environment to supplement theoretical and academic learning. They cited the closeness of the hospital to the student, the general low cost of
the system, and the merits for recruitment and retention of graduates as reasons
for a school that produced nurses within the hospital's own environment.

Opponents of the hospital-based system countered by arguing that the curriculum stressed training rather than education; the expenses were low only because costs were obscured and the students rendered a great deal of service in the
name of experience; and claims for recruitment and retention were highly exag-
gerated.

Over the years, pressure from accrediting bodies and state and national
nursing organizations has served to strengthen the curricula for all schools of
nursing. For the hospital schools, in particular, this meant a diminution of service
in favor of clinical practice under supervision, along with an increase in the number

of hours given to academic subjects, both general and professional. To some observers, these changes sufficed to meet the criticisms; to others, the alterations
were merely stopgaps to meet the surface problems. And for a third group, the
changes represented only further obstacles to solving the problems of nursing and
nursing manpower.

In their 1965 position paper on nursing education, the American Nurses'
Association stated unequivocally, "The education for all those who are licensed
to practice nursing should take place in institutions of higher education."[7] No
national schedule for implementation was given, but the state nurses' associations
were urged to work for accomplishment of the goals within their own areas. Reaction, and overreaction perhaps, was immediate; spokesmen were quick to rally to
the defense of the traditional system.

To the independent observer, there were a number of trends that pointed to
a restructuring of the educational patterns even before the ANA position paper.
For example, since the Second World War, there had been a marked reduction in
the number of hospital schools, with a corresponding increase in the number of
collegiate programs. True, these movements have been accelerated since 1965, but
their beginnings antedate the current controversies. Table 1 displays the changes
that have taken place over the past 15 years.

While these changes certainly reflect the efforts of organized nursing to
alter the institutional patterns of education, it is likely that the figures reflect the
changing patterns of public support and expectations for higher education as well.
Today, we are moving as a nation toward a norm of 14 years of general education,
following a trend in which first elementary, then secondary, and now postsecondary education is considered essential for the intellectual and vocational preparation
of citizens. In this light, just as the vocational high school has largely disappeared
in favor of the general secondary curriculum, so single-purpose, largely vocational
institutions are bowing to the competition of institutions that embody general

TABLE 1   NUMBER AND TYPE OF INSTITUTIONAL PROGRAMS FOR NURSING EDUCATION
IN THE UNITED STATES, 1953–1968

Year	Diploma	Associate Degree	Baccalaureate	More Than One Program
1953	926	*	95	104
1958	920	35	152	19
1963	857	102	177	6
1968	727	325	229	6

*No separate figure for AD programs

Source: *Facts About Nursing*

curriculum as well as vocational preparation. Nowhere is the effect of this public expectation seen more graphically than in the growth of the junior and community colleges in the United States. From a total of some 600 institutions in 1953, these schools increased to a new high of 890 in 1968. The replacement of hospital schools of nursing by collegiate institutions, then, follows the natural evolution of education within our culture.

The trends in our society, however, are not the only explanation for the demise of the hospital school. A survey by this commission of all those programs that had closed over the period of the last three years disclosed that internal problems had also taken their toll. Among those institutions that replied to the query, "What is the single most important factor responsible for your decision to close your program?" 52 percent cited lack of qualified faculty, while the remainder were almost evenly divided between problems of securing financing and securing students, aside from some miscellaneous reasons. Heads of harboring hospitals reported general agreement with these findings, placing perhaps more emphasis on the lack of qualified student applicants than on the matter of finances.

In an economic analysis of the supply of nurses, a research study supported by the U.S. Public Health Service, Altman found that students preferred programs that emphasized general education. This trend, in turn, increased the expenses of hospital schools and reduced the counterbalancing effects of rendered services.[8] He also noted a significant change in the occupational outlook of the female high school graduate which, when combined with other factors, tended to reduce the attractiveness of hospital-based programs.

When we submitted our conclusions on the predictable future patterns of nursing education to various agencies, we found very little disagreement. In one sampling, we found that 100 percent of the responding state hospital associations, state health departments, state boards of nursing, state nurses' associations, and state leagues for nursing agreed that the number of hospital nursing programs would be reduced in the years ahead. In the same survey, 88 percent of the state medical societies agreed. Between 80 and 100 percent of the same respondents felt that the greatest growth among institutions would come through the increase in junior or community college programs.

During our research we came to the conclusion that other questions needed to be explored on the desirability of these trends despite their powerful sweep. We were aware of the decline in the percentage of high school graduates going into nursing over the past few years, and had noted Altman's assertion that this development reflects a rejection, to some extent, of the hospital-based image. Our goal was to find out if there might be differing perceptions of the educational environment among nursing students themselves. To this end, a randomized, stratified sample of schools was drawn, and a Nursing Schools Environment Inventory

TABLE 2 SUMMARY OF COMPARISONS FROM THE NURSING SCHOOLS ENVIRONMENT
INVENTORY

| | Type of Institution | | |
Factor	Baccalaureate	Associate Degree	Diploma
General esteem	2*	1*	3
Academic enthusiasm	2*	1*	3
Extrinsic motivation	3	2*	1*
Breadth of interest	1	2*	3
Intrinsic motivation	1*	2*	3
Encapsulated training	3	1*	2*

prepared, similar to the Medical Schools Environment Inventory that had been used
in similar investigations by the Association of American Medical Colleges.* A total
of 283 schools was included in the sample, representing both sectional variation
and differences among types of preparatory programs. Approximately 5,300 students completed the questionnaires.

Six factors are assessed in the inventory: general esteem, academic enthusiasm, extrinsic motivation, intrinsic motivation, breadth of interest, and encapsulated training. With the possible exception of the last term, the factors are
generally self-explanatory. "Encapsulated training" refers to the degree to which
education is presented in packaged form to the students so that they must expend
their own efforts for interpretation and understanding.

While it must be emphasized that the instrument seeks only to assess perceptions, and not the validity of those perceptions, the results provide a revealing
look at student feeling. The collegiate students had significantly higher scores on
general esteem for their education, academic enthusiasm, breadth of interest, and
intrinsic motivation. The hospital school students were significantly higher in their
markings on extrinsic motivation, and, partially, on the factor of encapsulated
training. The ranking of the three kinds of institutions on these perceived educational factors is shown in Table 2; significant differences between ranks are indicated by asterisks.

By examining Table 2, we find that the baccalaureate students were highest
in perceived breadth of interest and intrinsic motivation, and lowest in perceived
extrinsic motivation and encapsulated training. All these differences might be in
directions that agree with common expectations. It may be surprising to note that
the associate degree students score highest on perceptions of general esteem and
academic enthusiasm. The perceptions of the diploma students tend to confirm a
number of the generalizations made about the differences between and among the
various institutions by those who seek to change the traditional patterns.

*A complete description and report on this study is included in the Appendix.

While students may have more positive perceptions about collegiate programs, there is still the final question concerning the relative effectiveness of the varying programs. Anecdotal comments abound that the associate degree graduates are not as competent as hospital school graduates. Some would even suggest that the hospital school nurses are superior to baccalaureate graduates who are steeped in theory but short on practice. We could certainly expect some differences to result merely from the varying lengths of the programs. A nurse with three years of preparatory training should differ from a graduate of a two- or four-year program. Likewise, we can expect a girl completing preparatory training at age 20 to react differently from a girl who graduates at age 22. Maturation is a crucial factor in education. To determine the extent and significance of some of these differences, our staff analyzed the results of the professional nursing examinations held in New York State in July of 1968. The findings are shown in Table 3.

While a written examination is only one sample of performance, the scores displayed in Table 3 suggest that some concerns about the emerging patterns of nursing education may be overdrawn. Note that the associate degree students placed lower on the average on each area of examination, but notice also that the diploma students scored lower on the average on each area than did the baccalaureate students. The most outstanding feature of the scores is the large overlap among all three programs. The indication is that variation in scores within one type of program is as great as variation between the three types of programs.

It can be expected that greater differences will emerge in areas like clinical performance when a two-year graduate is compared with an average three-year graduate. It seems likely, however, that differences within the programs will be at least as great as differences between them; any health care facility that employs nurses must take these variations into account in orientation and induction procedures.

For all these reasons, then—societal expectations, the attitudes of students, the growing availability of alternatives, and the measured outcomes of the programs—we believe that the future pattern of nursing education should be developed within the framework of our institutions for higher education. This would have the effect of redistributing the costs more equally among the populace and broadening the total base of support for programs in nursing education. Specifically, we recommend that:

> 1. *Each state have, or create, a master planning committee that will take nursing education under its purview, such committees to include representatives of nursing, education, other health professions, and the public, to recommend specific guidelines, means for implementation, and deadlines to ensure that nursing education is positioned in the mainstream of American educational patterns with its preparatory programs located in collegiate institutions.*

TABLE 3   RANGE OF INDIVIDUAL SCHOOL MEANS, AND MEANS OF ALL PROGRAMS. BY TYPE OF PROGRAM ON THE REGISTERED PROFESSIONAL NURSING EXAMINATIONS IN NEW YORK STATE, JULY 1, 1968

		Low	Mean	High
AD		397	447	533
DE	Medical	447	537	621
DI		394	516	606
AD		391	450	545
DE	Surgical	416	516	588
DI		324	504	569
AD		384	451	527
DE	Obstetric	454	525	628
DI		399	503	563
AD		370	443	519
DE	Pediatric	449	533	638
DI		377	514	608
AD		421	474	530
DE	Psychiatric	460	569	645
DI		392	507	595

Standard score 0   300   400   500   600   700   800

We recognize the outstanding contributions made by the hospital schools, and we are aware that a number of them possess most, if not all, of the requisites for accreditation as collegiate institutions in their own right. Therefore, we recommend that:

> 2. *Those hospital schools that are strong and vital, endowed with a qualified faculty, suitable educational facilities, and motivated for excellence be encouraged to seek and obtain regional accreditation and degree granting power.*

Our inquiries to the several regional accrediting associations have revealed differing degrees of interest in such a development. We strongly urge both the hospital schools that would seek accreditation and the accrediting associations to join in planning that could result in full recognition of those institutions that can meet the requirements.

True, not all the hospital schools have the structure, faculty, the facilities, or even the desire to pursue regional accreditation. To ensure their graduates of formal academic recognition and to provide them with full access to further educational opportunities, we suggest that these schools move quickly toward formalized arrangements with educational institutions that will permit the granting of degrees to the nurse graduates. In essence, this means that the educational institutions become responsible for the general and professional academic program, and the hospitals cooperate in providing the facilities for clinical instruction and practice. For this purpose, we recommend that:

> 3. *All other hospital schools of nursing move systematically and with dispatch (under the guidance of the state master planning committee), to effect interinstitutional arrangements with collegiate institutions so that:*
>
> a. *Graduates of the nursing preparatory program will receive an academic degree from the educational institution upon completion of their course of instruction;*
>
> b. *Joint planning takes place between the academic institution and the hospital on the articulation of instruction so that optimum use is made of clinical teaching facilities.*

In reality, this recommendation simply carries forward the growing number of interinstitutional compacts and brings them to a logical reformulation. Today, the majority of the hospital schools of nursing have some form of agreement for shared courses with one or more educational institutions. Unfortunately, many of these agreements do not call for courses that carry full academic credit and transferability. In these instances, it is the student who faces the hazards.

To ensure that one pitfall is not substituted for another under a new pattern, we also feel that the junior and senior colleges should eliminate any needless barriers to or between their programs. Capable nursing students should be able to continue their education with a minimum of difficulty. This does not mean that there should be blanket endorsement, nor does it mean that there might not be essential differences between the kinds of institutions that ought to survive. The burden, however, should rest on the institution to ensure that every opportunity for advanced learning is made available to each student. We recommend that:

> 4. *Junior and senior collegiate institutions cooperatively develop programs and curricula that will preserve the integrity of these institutions and their aims while facilitating the social and professional mobility of the nursing student.*

In urging this reorganization for nursing education, we are essentially recapitulating the recommendations of Brown,[9] Montag,[10] and Bridgman[11] together with those reported in studies conducted in North Dakota,[12] Alabama,[13] Illinois,[14] and Ohio.[15] These and other investigations have identified the need and the same general proposals for a transition in the patterns for nursing education. This commission feels that the recommendations are sound, and that the prospect of definitive state planning will lead to effective reordering. It would be wholly irresponsible to suggest the closing of hospital schools without planning for their adequate replacement by collegiate institutions. It is likewise irresponsible to cling to any pattern of education that shows increasing failure in meeting the needs and expectations of students, the profession, and the broad spectrum of parents and public. Change is implicit in human organization. That change can be planned and facilitated, rather than forced or subverted, is one of the strengths of this American society. North Dakota[16] has already demonstrated that a master plan for state-wide reorganization of nursing education can work. It is now incumbent on each of the other states to take the action to see that our institutions keep pace with accelerating health care needs.

PROBLEMS OF PREPARATORY INSTITUTIONS

When we interviewed the heads of harboring institutions for programs in nursing education to ascertain their analyses of the major problems in their own institutions, we found a broad area of consensus. The administrators singled out three predominant difficulties: shortage of qualified faculty (47 percent); lack of funds and financing (21 percent); and inadequate or outmoded facilities (13 percent). It seems obvious that these concerns may be relieved in part by the proposed reorganization of nursing education. At the same time, these problems have persisted for so long that we urge immediate steps to alleviate them.

Let us look for a moment at these difficulties and the possible solutions under the new patterns. In the first place, we believe that a broader base of support will develop for nursing education as the institutions change. In 1966, 82 percent of the hospital-controlled schools of nursing were privately supported;

in contrast, 91 percent of the junior or community college programs were supported by public funds.[17] While there are certainly hazards in public funding, there is the established pattern of massive public support for education through taxation, and this will accrue to nursing education as well.

One of the difficulties in financing nursing education in the past, however, has been the number and size of the programs. In the ten-year period from 1956 to 1966, the average number of students per school climbed from 103 to 114.[18] The average number of students per class is obviously much lower. This has meant the fractionating of support among a large number of programs, some of which are so small that they have less than 15 graduates per year. Likewise this situation has aggravated the difficulty of finding qualified faculty, and has often resulted in unnecessarily low student-faculty ratios.

In addition, it is generally agreed that the academic and clinical facilities for nursing education are inherently more expensive than for other courses of study. St. John's College in Cleveland, for example, found that the costs per student in nursing were approximately twice those for the student enrolled in the professional education sequence.[19]

Taken together, these conditions suggest that greater support should be provided to the institutions that are, and will be, engaged in nursing education. It is clear that scarce financial and faculty resources should be distributed through the most effective channels. To these ends, we recommend that:

> 5. *The state master planning committees be charged with drawing up a plan for each state to determine the number and minimum size of institutions to receive institutional and individual student aid; and*
>
> 6. *Small programs be terminated or consolidated into larger programs in order to reduce the per unit costs of education and in order to make better allocation of qualified faculty.*

For two reasons, we have declined to specify national standards for size of institution. In the first instance, the state committees are in a far better position to take into account local and institutional variations. Secondly, it is in no way the intent of this commission to arbitrarily reduce the number of openings for nursing applicants. In terminating smaller programs, and in redistributing resources, we feel that existing and developing institutions could readily enlarge the number of qualified applicants they accept. Thus, a program that is currently small may be encouraged and supported in its attempt to increase the number of students it serves. It would seem uneconomic, however, for an institution that consistently serves less than 25 nursing students per class to continue its preparatory program.

Aside from the expanded resources that could result from reorganization, nursing education does need substantial help from federal and state levels. In addition to scholarships and student loans, the institutions require aid in meeting operating costs that are far in excess of tuition income. This was recognized in the congressional authorization of $35,000,000 in the Health Manpower Act of 1968 for special projects and institutional grants. The administration request, however, was for $7,000,000 and eventually this was the amount appropriated.[20] While the situations are not analogous, it is interesting to note that in 1968 the federal government supplied over $98,000,000 to 69 American medical schools for faculty budgets through training and research grants.[21] This represented no less than one-third of the total faculty budget for these institutions. To help the institutions providing nursing education, we recommend that:

> 7. *Nursing education institutions be encouraged and given federal and state awards and support grants proportional to the number of students enrolled, such moneys to be used to defray the expenses of operation and expansion, and to provide salary support for qualified faculty.*

Along with institutional awards and grants for maintenance of programs, it seems particularly important in light of the administrators' views of the crucial need for support of new and/or modernized facilities that an increased program be initiated in this area. In 1968, the Health Manpower Act authorized $25,000,000 in construction grants for schools of nursing.[22] This could be viewed as an average of approximately $20,000 per school. Again, the actual appropriation sharply reduced the available amount. The final figure was $8,000,000, or approximately $6,400 per institution. Obviously, not every institution would be involved in construction in a given fiscal year, but the total available fund seems quite small when the estimated cost of one classroom building and its equipment for 360 students is in excess of $9,300,000. We recommend that:

> 8. *Federal and state grants for building and construction of facilities be sharply increased to up-date and enlarge laboratory and classroom areas. There should, however, be an effort made at each institution having multiple preparatory programs to encourage and plan joint, cooperative use of buildings, laboratories, etc.*

Money and proper planning can combine to solve most of the financial and facilities problems of nursing education. The shortage of qualified faculty is so widespread that one section of this report deals only with recommendations for the alleviation of this problem. As an interim measure, and perhaps as a useful approach for some time to come, we recommend that:

> 9. *Both state and regional committees explore the possibilities of sharing and increasing scarce faculty resources. A state, for example, might employ faculty*

through its university system to serve at several institutions for nursing education,
while both state and regional associations could develop programs for the profes-
sional advancement of current and future faculty personnel.

While it might seem that the state planning committees could be the best
source for suggestions on the shared use of faculty, the existing regional associations, such as the Upper Midwest Study group, the Southern Regional Education Board, the New England Board for Higher Education, and the Western Interstate Commission on Higher Education in Nursing, could enlarge the base for
cooperation, and could help supply the short-term answers, and perhaps long-
term solutions, to the persistent shortage of qualified nursing faculty.

Again, most of the recommendations designed to meet the critical problems
of educational institutions are neither new nor unique. At the state level, they are
anticipated by recommendations proposed in Illinois[23] and Massachusetts.[24] They
have similarly been anticipated by Brown[25] and other observers of the national
scene. Most important is that they have been accepted in principle as public policy
through the Nurse Training Act of 1964 and Title II of the Health Manpower Act of
1968. We strongly believe, however, that the actual financial appropriations must
meet the level of authorization. In addition, the authorization itself must be increased to match the needs of the large number of institutions required to prepare
enough nurses for our emerging health care delivery system.

ACCREDITATION OF EDUCATIONAL INSTITUTIONS

While perhaps not as dramatic as the problems of finance and building, one of
the vexing questions that nursing education must solve is accreditation. There
is a good deal of ferment on this subject nationwide. Many institutions of higher
education have serious questions on the need for separate accreditation of their
many academic programs by professional bodies and groups. This concern is
heightened by the variations in the forms and bodies that become involved in the
accreditation process. In particular, there is restlessness in the health fields over
the rising number of groups that seek recognition as the controlling agency for
specific accreditation practices. So deep is this division that one proposal has
already been offered for the establishment of an entirely new organization to conduct the accreditation of all educational programs in the health sciences, thus
offering a fresh start toward unravelling the jurisdictional disputes that mark
much of the effort in accreditation.[26]

As Selden suggests, "To meet fully its obligations both to its members and
society, a health professional association must have final responsibility for the

admission of its members."[27] He goes on to advise, however, that "they should provide in their structures for some greater representation of the public in order to assure that consideration will be given in their actions and policies to the public interest."[28]

Now seems to be an opportune time for nursing to review its accreditation policies in light of the recommendations for a changed institutional pattern in nursing education. In addition, the profession can take advantage of the growing awareness that some changed procedures might be of use to both the health professions and the educational institutions. Thus, we recommend that:

> 10. *A national committee be initiated by joint action of the American Nurses' Association and the National League for Nursing to study and make recommendations for future accrediting of nursing programs considering this commission's recommendations for changed institutional patterns and the several current proposals for altering accreditation procedures in other health fields.*

Membership on this committee should include representatives of the following: the accrediting group of the NLN, the Commission on Education of the ANA, the committee on accreditation of the AADN, state boards charged with accreditation, regional accrediting associations, institutions of higher education, the office of the United States Commissioner of Education, and the National Commission on Accrediting.

In addition to examining accreditation procedures, this committee would be wise to consider how public representation might be built into any proposal to ensure that "actions and policies [are in] the public interest."[29]

CURRICULAR NEEDS AND ARTICULATION

In the introduction to a proposed investigation of the curricular pattern in nursing, a researcher at the School of Nursing of the State University of Iowa notes, "Perhaps the most difficult problem which confronts the nursing education system, and the students who choose to prepare for nursing, is the absence of articulation between the various components of the system."[30] In the past, there have been many difficulties connected with the lack of congruency among the preparatory nursing programs. The graduate of a hospital school, for example, was likely to have difficulty in gaining credit for her completed course work when she applied for advanced placement in a collegiate program. From the college's point of view, however, there were extreme differences in quality among the hospital schools. Anything less than individual assessment of a student's placement might result in a "lack of fit" between the student and the faculty member's expectations of what had already been learned.

This lack of articulation is not a problem for the diploma school graduate alone. The graduate of a junior collegiate program finds difficulties in transferring to a baccalaureate program. The graduate of a liberal arts or science curriculum encounters problems in entering the nursing school without seemingly starting over for a second time. Of course, these conditions reflect real difficulties in the arrangement and order of course work. Nevertheless, they are problems that can waste time and energy, and they produce a deleterious influence on the concept of continuing personal advancement.

Such problems are not singular to nursing, though they are aggravated in this field because of the several kinds of preparatory programs. In recent years, there have been several efforts to define a core curriculum for the health sciences, a nucleus that might be shared by many of the professional schools. These studies, aimed at broadening the introduction to the health sciences, assume that there are some universals (things that all health professionals should know) as well as many alternatives (specialties that would obtain to one profession).

Consistent with such thinking, there have been national projects in the physical sciences, the biological sciences, and mathematics to organize and arrange curricula according to agreed universals, alternatives, and conceptual integrations. The results of these studies suggest that similar efforts for nursing might be well worthwhile. Of course, the institutions for nursing education have been active in the pursuit of curricular improvement. However, most of the attempts to study and implement new approaches have been limited to individual institutions—without a means for attacking the basic problem of articulation between varying kinds of preparatory schools. In a survey of individual and group reactions to our preliminary findings, a majority of our respondents concurred that few institutions in nursing were involved in large-scale curricular changes. Additionally, a high percentage felt that measurement and controlled evaluation were lacking in most of the curricular trials that were underway. There are obvious exceptions to these findings, and significant trials with novel curricular approaches are occurring at the universities of Colorado, Iowa, Kansas, and Purdue, and a number of other locations.

Our specific concern is that rigorous study of the curriculum transcend the objectives of any single institution. The focus should be on an integrated view of the needs of the proposed institutional patterns for future education of nurses. We do not suggest a single, monolithic approach to the development of a curriculum. Nursing has had experience with national curricula, including the standard curricula of 1917, 1927, and 1937. The profession is understandably reluctant to return to this track since a standard curriculum can serve as both a *minimum stand-*

ard and an impediment to innovation. The aim of a large-scale examination of the curriculum should be to ensure that each collegiate institution maintain its integrity, and a full measure of autonomy for experimentation, while striving at the same time to facilitate the educational, social, and professional mobility of the nursing student.

At the very least, this proposal calls for joint planning between the two collegiate levels that will comprise the future pattern of nursing education. To provide this planned articulation that will optimize student learning and facilitate career mobility, this commission recommends that:

> 11. *No less than three regional or interinstitutional committees be funded for the study and development of the nursing curriculum to develop educational objectives, universals, alternatives, and sequences for instruction. These committees should seek to specify appropriate levels of general and specialized learning for the different types of educational institutions.*

It is the firm conviction of this commission that nursing alone can determine the objectives, content, and sequences of its professional curriculum. In the suggested studies, however, we urge the involvement of consultants and advisors from other disciplines (as did medicine in the Endicott House Summer Study on Medical Education[31]), including specialists from the social, physical, and natural sciences. It is one of the great challenges of nursing that its curriculum spans so wide a range of academic disciplines. At the same time, this broad spectrum offers a tremendous opportunity for obtaining the counsel of many specialists on the vital aspects of their field in relation to nursing students.

At the risk of repeating thoughts that most nursing educators have long espoused, we urge that the general public be made aware of the basic assumptions that underlie any of the curricular proposals that emerge from the several study groups. These basic assumptions should include:

> a. *The acceptance, as a core value of our American culture, that education should be an open-ended process and that access to enlarged opportunities is a right of every individual;*
> b. *As a corollary, care must be taken in curricular planning to avoid unnecessary impediments before or between collegiate programs in nursing that would inhibit the orderly transfer and acceptance of qualified individuals who wish to pursue higher career goals.*

In the past, because of the confusion over the varied preparatory programs, nursing education acquired a reputation for difficult transfer and advanced placement. It is imperative that the profession face this problem and make every effort to ensure that the individual student is given opportunity that matches ability and motivation.

Without encroaching on the deliberations of the curriculum study committees, the commission would suggest, as a result of the staff search of the literature as well as the many discussions and site visits, that two propositions might be investigated. One of these is the development of course concentrations for the emerging practice of distributive nursing care in addition to the sequences that currently prepare nurses for episodic care facilities. The second suggestion is the possible development of an integrated health core curriculum that could serve as an introduction to the mutually dependent roles of the health professions.

Following the development of the several curriculum plans, the commission recommends that:

> 12. *Federal, state, and private funds be invested in a small number of grants for the specific purpose of demonstrating, testing, and evaluating the proposed curricula emanating from the study committees.*

The benefits from the curriculum studies can come only when new patterns are implemented. It is very important, however, that these proposals be evaluated and measured at the outset so that good features might be retained and poor ones deleted. Based on study and analysis, we might hope for varied but useful approaches to nursing education and to effective articulation among the institutions involved.

GRADUATE STUDY AND FACULTY DEVELOPMENT

The public has been sensitized to the need to prepare more nurses. As indicated earlier in this chapter, one of the prime problems faced by the educational institutions is the shortage of qualified faculty to handle current, let alone expanded, class loads. This situation requires a delicate balancing act on the part of planners. The number of graduate and advanced students must be increased, but a proliferation of graduate programs could heighten the scarcity of faculty and depress the quality of education. It is essential that strong graduate programs be enlarged before new (and perhaps marginal) ones are established. We recommend that:

> 13. *The state master planning committee for nursing education be particularly concerned that the number of graduate programs in nursing be consistent with human and economic resources, and that the inauguration or expansion of weak programs not be permitted.*

Priority in providing financial support for graduate programs in nursing should go for three particular types of preparation: for individuals who intend to take faculty positions in institutions for preparatory nurse training; for individuals intent on becoming master clinicians, i.e., nurses capable of providing excellent direct patient care while serving as role models for nursing students; and for persons wishing to specialize in the organization and delivery of nursing services, particularly for the emerging systems of health care. To ensure that these three simultaneous and urgent needs are met, we recommend that:

14. *The Congress continue and expand such programs as the Health Manpower Act to:*
a. *Provide educational loans to nurses pursuing graduate degrees with provision for part or whole forgiveness based on subsequent years of teaching;*
b. *Provide postmaster and postdoctoral fellowships and traineeships for nursing faculty and master clinicians to permit added professional development and continuing reorientation to changing practice and developing health care delivery systems;*
c. *Provide earmarked funds for faculty members of schools of nursing to enable them to obtain additional formal academic preparation equal to that required for regular appointment to faculty posts in collegiate institutions. These funds should have similar forgiveness features based on years of continuing service.*

The last provision above is based on NLN data supported by our own staff findings indicating that one out of five current faculty members in nursing has less than a baccalaureate education, and three out of five have no more than a baccalaureate degree. Of course, there are strong regional and institutional variations, but it seems obvious that we need to direct the development of faculty—to enhance their own future and the quality of their instruction.

In addition to financial aid for present and future nursing faculty, imaginative steps must be taken now and for some time to come to ensure the most effective utilization of the qualified individuals who are available. In recommendation 9, we suggested the joint appointment of faculty members to more than one institution, under either state or regional auspices. The Center for Nursing Education in Spokane, Washington, is an arresting example of such interinstitutional cooperation through joint faculty appointment and shared finances. A number of nursing schools have developed a high degree of cooperation with other departments and professional schools (particularly those of medicine, education, and public health) in providing relevant courses, and in the shared use of classrooms, laboratories, and other facilities. The need for improvement remains, however, in the joint use and planning of institutional resources. As a minimum first step, nursing should make every effort to avoid duplication of courses, sequences, and faculty appointments that are available (or properly developed) in other schools or departments, or provided through core teaching. Such a suggestion flies in the face of the strong desire to be wholly independent; it is essential, however, if nursing is to realize the economic use of resources.

In addition to the benefits of shared faculty and facilities, we urge the exploration of new educational technologies that can enhance learning effectiveness and efficiency. This commission recommends that:

15. *Federal, state, and private funds be made available to nursing institutions:*

a. *In the form of small research grants or contracts to assess and evaluate the effectiveness of new media and technology for nursing education and to disseminate the results;*

b. *In the form of grants and stipends to support short-term workshops to acquaint faculty members with new media and instructional materials;*

c. *In the form of institutional grants or matching funds to permit the purchase and installation of media systems and the required technicians to maintain and operate them;*

d. *In the form of demonstration grants to develop a limited number of centers so that faculty members may visit and have "actual" experience with these new media and materials.*

Without any denigration of the quality of traditional instruction, there is abundant evidence that new media and technology can be effectively applied to the teaching of the health sciences in general and to nursing in particular.[32] It has been determined, for example, that programmed instruction for nursing students can result in higher achievement coupled with more efficient learning.[33] In addition, computer-aided instruction, simulation, multimedia presentations, and technological systems can probably have a profound effect on the current lack of qualified faculty. Moreover, these additions to the instructional techniques are no longer mere promises. Beginning research has verified their utility for nursing, but much more inquiry, and far more development work, is required.

A final area to be considered in the examination of advanced and graduate study is that of doctoral programs. In 1967, there were only 209 nurses known to be enrolled in doctoral programs. There were 19 known doctorates awarded that year to nurses. The staggering impact of these figures is alleviated, in part, because some unknown number of nurses are working in, or have graduated from, doctoral programs in arts and sciences, education, and public health. It is most difficult to assign numbers to these advanced graduates, but it is generally accepted in the profession that the total is still small.

There are evident needs for graduate programs at the master's level to produce faculty and master clinicians *now* for unfilled positions. Yet, it must be recognized that doctoral holders are essential both to produce the finished graduate student at the master's level and to generate the research that is so crucial—the research that this commission has identified as the only clear means for eventually solving the long-term problems of the profession. But research requires competence, and in our particular system of education, this competence is developed only in the doctoral programs of the various academic disciplines. In our inquiries to specialists in nursing, medicine, and the other health fields concerning the lacks in our current system, we found almost unanimous agreement that "most nurse faculty members lack research competence." Again, this is a statement of common experience. It also describes a situation that must be altered. At the same time, we suggest that there must be a series of graded accelerations in the enlargement of doctoral programs in nursing because the profession simply does not have the numbers of qualified faculty to permit a marked jump in enrollment. This commission recommends that:

> 16. *Federal, state, and private funds be extended to support a limited number of institutions to establish or expand doctoral programs in nursing science. These programs should focus on developing research capabilities for the study of nursing practice and nursing education, and should undertake the specification and development of nursing theory and knowledge.*

Coincident with the commitment to increase and improve the doctoral programs in nursing science, funds must be provided to support the basic and applied research into both nursing practice and nursing education. In the previous chapter, we enunciated a recommendation for inquiry into the outcomes of nursing practice (see Chapter Four, pp. 84 to 86); it is likewise essential that we provide for scientific inquiry into the content, objectives, and methodologies of nursing education. We recommend that:

> 17. *The federal Division of Nursing, the National Center for Health Services Research and Development, other governmental agencies, and private foundations provide research funds and contracts for basic and applied research into the nursing curriculum, articulation of educational systems, instructional practices, facilities design, etc., so that the most functional, effective, and economic approaches are taken in the education and development of future nurses.*

With the development of more knowledge about the nature and content of nursing education, we can gain better control over the factors that contribute to attrition and low student achievement.

INSTITUTIONAL ADMISSION AND RETENTION

In the foregoing discussion of institutional patterns, we pointed out that individual students encounter difficulty, and sometimes hardship, in transferring from one program to another. While the proposals for the new pattern of nursing education will facilitate this process, educational specialists recognize that there remain individual differences in experience and accomplishment that are not reflected in accumulated course hours and grades. To ensure both personalized treatment and proper placement within programs, we recommend that:

18. *The institutions for nursing education develop new approaches to the matter of admissions, including:*

a. *Development of both written and performance examinations to assess the quality of prior nursing experience and practice for the purposes of credit and advanced placement;*

b. *Development of achievement, placement, and diagnostic examinations in academic subjects to provide credit and proper placement of individuals within instructional programs.*

While various educational institutions and disciplines have used testing procedures as a basis for awarding both credit and advanced placement, we recognize that the emphasis on this approach to individual admission and assignment has received increased attention in the past five years. Propelled by the development of advanced placement tests for talented high school students, interest has been aroused in the development of tests that will aid in recognizing achievement by a wide range of individuals through sources other than traditional classroom work. New York State, for example, has developed a number of college course equivalency tests through which a person can demonstrate competence in a field— competence that may have been gained through individual reading, study, or other nonstandard approaches. Of late, a number of these tests have been developed in areas of nursing study. Early experience with these examinations indicates that a high percentage of applicants are able to demonstrate acceptable competence on the tests. Much more needs to be done in the development and refinement of these tests, and individual institutions will undoubtedly vary in their approach. However, the trend toward greater individualization seems one of the truly encouraging developments in educational practice.

Related to the trends in admission and placement is the matter of student retention. Approximately one out of three entering students in nursing withdraws before graduation. This figure varies somewhat among institutions, and within geographic areas, but remains a relatively constant diminution factor. While a number of investigations have attempted to determine the factors related to withdrawal, little has been demonstrated in the area of reliable measurement. Obviously, more needs to be learned about this phenomenon. The commission recommends that:

19. *To decrease student withdrawals and academic failures, nursing preparatory institutions:*

a. *Study their application procedures, academic advising, and student completion data for the purpose of developing better selection and counseling;*

b. *Investigate the development of more individualized programs of instruction that require accomplishment of curricular objectives, but permit variance in student rate of learning and in the number of courses taken at any one time.*

While it is essential that we develop better information on selection and retention, it may be possible that more individual variation within the academic program could have a salutary effect on increased student completion of the nursing sequence. It might be worth mentioning that lock-step programs in all academic fields have debilitating effects, both on students who could move more rapidly and on students who should progress more slowly. Growing capacity to allow the student to learn at his own rate can mean acceleration for the talented as well as deceleration for the capable but less rapid learners.

CONTINUING AND IN-SERVICE EDUCATION

In our survey of nursing organizations, medical societies, and health management representatives, we found almost unanimous agreement on the growing necessity for increased and improved programs in the fields of continuing and in-service education. The respondents were in close accord in their feeling that technological advances, altered aspects of practice and care delivery, and the general social changes in the health professions and the larger culture would combine to make life-long learning a practical necessity. For this reason, it is essential that all educational programs in nursing stress the professional responsibility of the nurse for his or her own continual learning. Never before was the appellation "terminal program" less meaningful, or perhaps more dangerous. Constant concern for being up-to-date must characterize all types and levels of nursing.

While the responsibility for continued learning must reside with the individual, we strongly urge that more effective aids be supplied to all health personnel in the future to help meet the accelerating changes in health practice We recommend that:

20. *The state master planning committee for nursing education identify one or more institutions to be responsible for regional coverage of continuing education programs for nurses within that area, and further that:*

a. *Federal and state funds be utilized to plan and implement continuing education programs for nursing on either a statewide or broader basis (as suggested by the current interstate compacts for higher education); and*

b. *In the face of changing health roles and functions, and the interdependence of the health professions, vigorous efforts be taken to have continuing education programs jointly planned and conducted by interdisciplinary teams.*

The same reasoning that suggests a need for better continuing education leads to the consideration of in-service education. By definition, this area is located closer to the point of application and includes the instructional practices of the institution or facility. Historically, nursing has played a major role in in-service education, both for its own personnel and for the auxiliaries, aides, and other kinds of personnel employed in health institutions. At the same time, the entire commitment to in-service education has been characterized by inadequate support and insufficient personnel. Of the more than 7,000 hospitals in the United States, for example, no more than 300 have a professional training specialist to direct their in-service program. All too frequently, responsibility has devolved upon nursing service in the absence of any specific plan for implementation. While nursing should continue to contribute its talents in cooperation with the other professions, we recommend that:

> 21. *Health care facilities, including hospitals, nursing homes, and other institutions, either individually or collectively through joint councils, provide professional training staffs to supervise and conduct in-service training and provide released time, facilities, and organizational support for the presentation of in-service nursing education as well as that for other occupations.*

It is reasonable to expect that the regional medical programs and comprehensive health planning agencies will make a signal contribution to both continuing and in-service education in the coming years. It will be the responsibility of the individual nurse, and the professional organizations representing the nurses, to extract as much benefit as possible from these emerging forces.

FINANCING OF THE RECOMMENDATIONS

Traditionally, nursing education has been largely a matter of private financing, but with a marked trend toward higher levels of public support. In fiscal 1969, for example, the federal government appropriated $6,500,000 for nursing scholarships. For the year ending June 30, 1970, the administration requested $12,000,000, and the final appropriation for that period was $7,178,000.

Scholarship funds, however, may not be the most critical single element in the list of priorities. Institutional support and construction grants, advanced traineeships for nursing research and faculty development, as well as grants and contracts for research are necessities in the development of nursing practice and the enhancement of nursing careers. In authorizing funds for institutional construction, Congress specified $25,000,000; the administration, however, requested only eight. Thirty-five million dollars was authorized for special projects and institutional grants; only $7,000,000 was requested. Other authorizations were subjected to similar reductions. In all these instances, the administration is necessarily attempting to balance calls on available funds that are far in excess of money available. However, the effect on nursing and the capacity of the United States to attain significant goals in health care is most unfortunate.

To provide funds for research and for institutional support for the educational programs in nursing, we must begin now to increase the level of public and private support. In the period from 1960 through 1968, federal support for nursing multiplied over seven times. Yet, total federal support for professional nursing in 1968 was less than double that provided for practical nursing and auxiliaries. It would seem that the minimum level of federal support for the immediate future would be in terms of the already authorized levels of expenditure, with state governments providing appropriate supplements in such critical areas as construction and institutional grants. Private funds could supply aid for quality research and educational innovation. We recommend that:

> 22. *Federal, regional, state, and local governments adopt measures for the increased support of nursing research and education. Priority should be given to construction grants, institutional grants, advanced traineeships, and research grants and contracts. Further, we recommend that private funds and foundations support nursing research and educational innovations where such activities are not publicly aided. We believe that a useful guide for the beginnings of such a financial aid program would be in the amounts and distribution of funds authorized by Congress for fiscal 1970, with proportional increases from other public and private agencies.*

While the congressional authorization provides scholarship funds—and we recommend their retention—we recognize that the increased share of public support for nursing education has somewhat reduced the need for individual financial aid at the preparatory level. In fact, many scholarships do not meet the institutional costs involved in educating a nurse. Most educational institutions find their costs far in excess of their income from tuition. It is for this reason that we emphasize a program of institutional and construction grants to offset the costs of operation.

To provide needed funds for research and educational support, we propose expenditures in the range of those authorized by Congress in the Health Manpower Act, or $110 to 125 million in fiscal 1971. This figure would represent a modest part of the total budget for health, education, and welfare, which in 1969 was estimated at $50 billion. It is less than three times the support level currently provided for practical nurses and auxiliaries, and is only one-eighth the current level of federal support for medical education and research. We should note that, in comparison to the medical field, nursing has four times as many students and ten times the number of individual schools.

The minimum figure recommended just matches the estimated 1969 appropriation of $110 million for the Peace Corps. In contrast to the estimated outlays for other social purposes, such as the $4.344 billion spent on highways and $421 million for removal of surplus commodities, our recommendation would seem to represent a modest sum. Considering the importance of our health care system and the significance of nursing in that system, a public investment of this magnitude would seem to be fully justified.

Following the categories employed by Congress in the Health Manpower Act, we propose that the following amounts be appropriated:

Category	Minimum Level	Desirable Level
Construction grants	$25,000,000	$30,000,000
Scholarships	12,000,000	15,000,000
Loans	20,000,000	20,000,000
Special and institutional grants	35,000,000	38,000,000
Advanced training	15,000,000	18,000,000
Research	3,000,000	4,000,000
Total	$110,000,000	$125,000,000

This commission considers the minimum figures to represent irreducible sums required for nursing to meet the national demands for health care in the immediate future. More properly, the amounts should be viewed as a base for expanded appropriations. Nursing education, for example, now has more than 10,000 individual faculty members who do not possess postbaccalaureate training.[34] It will require six years at the minimum fund level to erase this professional deficit. Moreover, Yett has shown convincingly that funds in the federal formula for institutional grants do not offer an incentive to schools to expand their enrollment, and, indeed, often lead to a discouraging point of diminishing return.[35]

It is possible that some of the proportions among the categories listed should be readjusted over the years. Experience with the loan and scholarship features of the total appropriation might well be used as indices for future construction program monies and funds for other categories.[36] Relatedly, the proportion of funds for scholarships might be altered by the shift from privately supported hospital schools to publicly supported collegiate preparatory programs. The likelihood of this seems a bit remote. Most nursing students come from families in middle and lower socioeconomic levels. Successful efforts to attract more disadvantaged persons into nursing would certainly offset the gains received from greater public support of nursing institutions.

It must be observed that the sums authorized in the Health Manpower Act were developed in light of the long-range analyses of the Surgeon General's Consultant Group, the Program Review Committee for the Nurse Training Act, and the National Advisory Council on Nurse Training, which included public representatives as well as health professionals and government officials. Moreover, the figures proposed do not represent notably large increases over recent federal appropriations for professional nursing. These were $80.6 and $81.4 million in 1967 and 1968, respectively. It would seem that our figures are based on a factual, reasoned analysis of the minimum levels of federal support needed today. They must certainly be enlarged in the future.

There must also be increased supplementary aid from the states. We are becoming painfully aware of the critical needs for health care and its delivery throughout the country, but we have yet to face up to the monetary requirements that result. While each of the states has certainly provided some support for nursing, it is insufficient to meet the critical needs for construction, institutional grants, and faculty-student aid. In 1966–67, state governments contributed $142 million to the support of medical schools—an amount greater than our commission's request for federal funds for nursing. Amounts varied, and the terms of support differed from state to state, including the channeling of some funds through the regional compacts for higher education.[37] Similar state or regional programs must be undertaken in nursing to ensure that sufficient numbers of qualified individuals are available to meet the deepening health problems of the nation.

It is likely that the private sector of the economy—the foundations, funds, and private philanthropists—can make its greatest contribution to nursing through the support of research and innovation. Through emphasis on developing greater knowledge about nursing practice, education, and care delivery, there is every promise that a more capable and more responsive profession will emerge. There will always be a need for private funds, and, of course, these should be directed to the areas for which governmental funds may not be available.

With continued acceleration in federal support, and with proportional increases in assistance from other governmental and private sources, the financial problems of nursing could be alleviated (though not fully solved). With the levels of support suggested here, however, we would have the capability of getting on with the conduct of research and educational development that are required to bring nursing up-to-date and into partnership in the delivery of quality health care. We believe that nursing, given that opportunity, can generate more increased support for itself in future years.

FOOTNOTES

1. Goldmark, J. *Nursing and Nursing Education in the United States.* New York: The Macmillan Company. 1923.
2. Brown, E. L. *Nursing for the Future.* New York: Russell Sage Foundation. 1948.
3. Montag, M. *Education of Nursing Technicians.* New York: G. P. Putnam's Sons. 1951.
4. Bridgman, M. *Collegiate Education for Nursing.* New York: Russell Sage Foundation. 1953.
5. Goldmark, J., *op. cit.,* pp. 194–195.
6. Brown, E. L., *op. cit.,* See recommendations concerning "Distinguished Hospital Schools."
7. American Nurses' Association. "Educational Preparation for Nurse Practitioners and Assistants to Nurses: A Position Paper." New York: American Nurses' Association. 1965. p. 5.
8. Altman, S. H. "The Structure of Nursing Education and Its Impact on Supply." Preliminary draft of a report developed under U.S.P.H.S. Contract No. PH 108-67-204, "Economic Analysis of the Supply of Nurses." The preliminary draft was kindly supplied to our staff by Professor Altman for their use in analysis. The final report will be publicly available.
9. Brown, E. L., *op. cit., passim.*
10. Montag, M., *op. cit., passim.*
11. Bridgman, M., *op. cit., passim.*
12. North Dakota Joint Committee on Nursing Needs and Resources. "The Need to Know." Minneapolis, Minnesota: Upper Midwest Nursing Study, 1969, *passim.*
13. Alabama Board of Nursing. "Assessment of Nursing Education in Alabama, 1968." Montgomery, Alabama: Alabama Board of Nursing. 1968. See recommendations, p. 22.
14. Illinois Study Commission on Nursing. "Nursing in Illinois: An Assessment and a Plan, 1968–1980." Chicago, Illinois: Illinois Study Commission on Nursing. 1968. See recommendation No. 25, p. 13.
15. Joint Committee on Nursing Education. "Projected Needs for Nursing Education in Ohio." Columbus, Ohio: Ohio State Nurses' Association. 1964., *passim.*
16. North Dakota Joint Committee on Nursing Needs and Resources, *op. cit.*
17. American Nurses' Association. *Facts About Nursing, 1968 Edition.* New York: American Nurses' Association. 1968. p. 106.
18. *Ibid.,* p. 105.
19. Personal Communication, October, 1969.
20. "Aid to Nurse Education Lower in Proposed Federal Budget." *American Journal of Nursing.* 69:3:445. March, 1969.
21. "Datagrams: Federal Grant Support of Faculty Salaries." *Journal of Medical Education.* 44:6:551–552. June, 1969.
22. "Aid to Nurse Education Lower in Proposed Federal Budget." *op. cit.*
23. Illinois Study Commission on Nursing., *op. cit.*
24. Malone, M. F. "Study of Nursing Education in the Commonwealth of Massachusetts Prepared for the Board of Higher Education." Boston, Massachusetts: Board of Higher Education. 1968. *mimeo.*
25. Brown, E. L., *op. cit.*
26. Selden, W. K. "Just One Big Happy Family." *Health Alliance.* 1:2:8. September, 1969.

27. *Ibid.,* p. 7.

28. *Ibid.,* p. 8.

29. *Ibid.*

30. "A Design for Articulation: A New Approach to Increasing Opportunities for Baccalaureate Nursing Education." University of Iowa College of Nursing. Undated. *mimeo.,* p. 1. This draft of a proposal for the funding of a curricular study was provided to the study staff through the kindness of Dean Laura C. Dustan.

31. Cope, O. and J. Zacharias. *Medical Education Reconsidered.* Philadelphia: J. B. Lippincott Company. 1966.

32. Lysaught, J. P. "Studies on the Use of Programmed Instruction in Nursing Education." in Dunn, W. R. and C. Holroyd (Eds.) *Aspects of Educational Technology, II.* London: Methuen and Company, Ltd. 1969.

33. —— "Self-Instruction in Nursing Education: The Impact of Technology on Professional Curricula." *Educational Technology.* 9:7. July, 1969.

34. American Nurses' Association., *op. cit.,* p. 12.

35. Yett, D. E. "The Nursing Shortage and the Nursing Training Act." *Hospital Topics.* 44:6:29. June, 1966.

36. *Ibid.,* p. 28.

37. "Datagrams: State Aid to Medical Schools." *Journal of Medical Education.* 44:10:1000–1001. October, 1969.

SIX
FINDINGS AND RECOMMENDATIONS ON NURSING CAREERS

Unquestionably the supply of nurse manpower is a key element in the provision of adequate health care in the United States. If we have a shortage of nurse practitioners today, there is every assurance that the problem will deepen as new treatments and new preventive measures are introduced. The fact is that we have lived so long with nursing scarcity that we have evolved two traditional "solutions" for the problem that we repeat year after year. First, there is the annual campaign to multiply the number of nursing students. Second, there is the companion effort to increase the categories of helping personnel, i.e., practical nurses, nurse aides, attendants, and orderlies.

If nothing else, the continued shortage of nurses should indicate the shortcomings of these traditional methods. It would seem that what we have done for so long is to attack only the manifestations of the problem without getting at the root causes. Improved manpower planning, to cite one new approach, might remove some of the crisis elements that appear in urgent and repeated appeals for more nursing students; at the same time, it could help us identify more definitive needs in terms of types and numbers of personnel required to assure optimum care.

In the same vein, we must reexamine the basic satisfactions of the profession. The nursing shortage is underscored dramatically by both the number of inactive licensed nurses and the high rate of turnover experienced in most health agencies.

Finally, the profession must evaluate the current emphasis on quantity of nursing service to the near exclusion of quality considerations. The capability required of today's nurse practitioners makes it mandatory that prospective students be recruited through careful screening. Health personnel are not mere hands; and the growing complexity of care should serve to deemphasize our concern with numbers alone.

In this area of our study, we examined the factors that are central to the supply of nursing services, the enhancement of careers in nursing, and the assurance of competence in nursing practice. Specifically, our investigation explored the ways to plan for nursing careers, retain qualified practitioners, recruit prospective students, develop new sources of manpower, streamline licensing procedures, and strengthen the organizations that serve nurses.

Our staff utilized three major sources for information. First, we conducted an exhaustive study of state, regional, and national investigations into nursing manpower and personnel. In particular, these documents were examined for their data on influences in the supply of nursing personnel, trends in nursing careers, and satisfactions of continued practice in nursing.

Secondly, we reviewed the general literature in the field, including both journal and research articles, for information on regional health planning, utilization of personnel, innovations in personnel policy to enhance careers, and various incentive and compensation systems.

Finally, the on-site visits by the staff gave us the opportunity to explore the issues, and various proposals for dealing with them, with a broad range of specialists. These included nurses, physicians, health managers, business and industrial personnel experts, insurers' representatives, and a number of consumers' representatives.

PLANNING FOR NURSING CAREERS

The shortage in the supply of nurses has been discussed at length in Chapter Three[1] and again, in terms of the nursing role, in Chapter Four.[2] However, when it comes to enhancing careers through improved planning and manpower development, there would seem to be two areas that require attention. The first is the extension of nursing's voice in planning operations; the second is the development of more sophisticated approaches for the delineation of manpower requirements.

While it is impossible to foresee all the responsibilities that will be thrust at the profession in the future, there is ample evidence that we need to bring nurses more directly into today's health planning operations. Until recently, the National Advisory Commission on Health Manpower had not a single nurse among its members, and only one nurse on any of its seven specialized panels. Recently this oversight has been recognized by some health planners, and a number of states have taken steps to appoint nurses to comprehensive health planning agencies.[3] At the national level, also, corrective action has taken place. Two years ago, the American Hospital Association was reorganized so that nursing now has a voice in all areas of its activities. In a related development, the Joint Commission on Accreditation of Hospitals, which still has no formal representation from nursing, obtained a review of its standards by the American Nurses' Association—a preliminary step toward a more meaningful relationship.[4]

It is evident that nurses must be involved in overall planning for health care. Every proposal for changed institutional patterns, staffing, and treatment has direct effects on the nursing profession. And those who seek to make the career more attractive recognize that nurses need a voice in the determination of their future responsibilities. Moreover, nursing has its own specialized knowledge that represents a needed input into decision-making about health care procedures. At a time when "community participation" is a potent force, it is unrealistic to deprive the health community of nursing's contribution to health planning. We recommend that:

> 1. *Nurses be appointed to, and hold full membership in, groups involved in health manpower planning at all governmental and regional levels.*

At the same time, we commend the federal Division of Nursing and the professional associations within nursing for the on-going studies they have generated on manpower needs. We urge them to continue this work. It is essential, however, that the regional and local decisions that will have crucial repercussions for nursing practice and careers be developed with the full participation of nursing representatives, from initial discussions and planning to final decision-making.

The inclusion of nurses on planning bodies can have a salutary effect on the other problem related to planning and nursing careers: the recruitment of nurses for specific care areas. Too frequently, manpower projections are couched in terms of needed numbers of "registered nurses" and "other personnel." The very changes in roles and functions of nursing, along with the changes in health practice and technology generally, emphasize the shallowness of such an approach. A total number of registered nurses, for example, does not differentiate between the number of professionals needed for episodic, as opposed to distributive, care activities. Within the developing structure of functional expertise, some discrimination is required in terms of staff nurse, clinical nurse, and master clinician. It seems almost trite to say that only nurses can be instrumental in translating general figures into specific requirements for the numbers, levels, and specialized skills needed among practitioners. Only nurses, in concert, of course, with other health professions, can define the emerging specialties to ensure that planning is made feasible in day-to-day operations. This commission recommends that:

> 2. *Manpower planning in nursing be premised on the concept that nursing is primarily a clinical practice directed to the care of people. An adequate supply of practitioners, plus the effective and efficient utilization of this resource, requires more than general planning projections.*
> a. *Planning should take into account the developing types and levels of nursing, including the pattern of staff, clinical, and master clinician nurse, and the functional distribution of nurses into episodic and distributive fields.*
> b. *Planning should include the categories of non-nursing personnel (clerks, housekeepers, receptionists, registrars) required to free nurses from tasks not related to the direct care of people.*
> c. *Planning should also take into account those categories of health workers required to provide routine personal and therapeutic services—those currently known as practical nurses, aides, auxiliaries, attendants.*

It is critical to the planning process that guidelines be altered in light of research into nursing practice and innovations in organization and technology. Planning, by definition, should be a projection, not a recapitulation. It is essential that planning facilitate change and improvement rather than serve as a report on the *status quo.*

RETENTION OF QUALIFIED PRACTITIONERS

While planning can help us to determine the number and kinds of practitioners we will require, it is vital that we undertake immediate steps to reduce the attrition rate in the profession. The potential for solving our manpower problems through improved retention is quite promising. A projection by the federal Division of Nursing, for example, indicates that a 1 percent increase in nurse retention could expand the supply of practitioners in 1976 by 46,000 nurses—a figure as large as the anticipated number of nursing graduates that year.[5]

Inactive nurses constitute a great potential. Almost half of all graduate nurses are not employed in nursing at the present time; yet half these individuals retain licenses. There is evidence that these nurses represent some elasticity in supply because we find increases in both the number of part-time nurses and the percentage of married nurses returning to employment.[6]

Unfortunately, the gains in retention (or reactivation) are largely offset by the losses in turnover. Nationally, registered nurse practitioners represent a turnover rate of 70 percent.[7] This means that during a 12-month period, the *average* facility must replace seven out of every ten nurses. Some institutions experience a 100 percent turnover rate or more, i.e., no less than one replacement for every nurse employed. At an estimated cost of $420 per replacement, the financial burden is high, but the costs in terms of work organization and care delivery are even higher.[8] So frustrating, and so pervasive, are these problems that some observers suggest that our national preoccupation with a nursing shortage stems as much from the turnover pattern as from any absolute lack of practitioners.

These phenomena—inactivity and turnover—are not solely a consequence of the dominantly female composition of the profession. There are characteristic periods of employment interruption due to marriage, childbirth, and child-rearing. Yet in contrast to other "female" occupations, nursing seems to display inherent weakness. For example, the national rate of turnover among teachers, another predominantly female force, is less than 20 percent each year.[9]

Certainly, there are strains and distress inherent in constant contact with the ill and injured that distinguish nursing from other occupations. But nursing in general exhibits behaviors that are characteristic of what Argyris describes as "unhealthy organizations."[10] Specifically, he mentions frequency of turnover as an indication of flight from an unhappy situation, followed by increasing frustration as the individual finds the next job—and the next—no different. It seems conceivable that many nurses find their assignments equally unsatisfying wherever they go.

In Chapter Four, we considered the need for providing nurses with continued opportunities to remain in practice. Many studies have shown that nurses' intrinsic satisfaction with their career relates positively to their direct involvement in care.[11] Our recommendations to develop a series of career levels in nursing practice emanate from our findings that link individual nursing satisfaction with continuation of nursing practice. Unfortunately, many of the trends in the past have constituted pressures to remove nurses from direct patient care.

It would be unrealistic to overlook the impact of economics on the retention and reactivation of nurses. Despite recent notable gains in the starting salaries of those entering nursing, there continues to be little financial reward or incentive for maintaining a career in practice. In the recently published salary standards of the state nurses' associations, for example, there are modest—even meager— differentials proposed between beginning and experienced nurses.[12] An inquiry conducted by the American Hospital Association in 1969 disclosed that 75 percent of the community hospitals in the United States pay their nurse practitioners less than $7,500 per year.[13] These are hardly the kinds of salary schedules that could offer an incentive to continue in the profession—certainly not as a direct purveyor of patient care.

A number of forward-looking health facilities have already established levels for clinical practitioners that essentially anticipate the recommendations advanced by the commission.[14] The capabilities that the individual must demonstrate to earn promotion in levels are clearly spelled out, as are any appropriate subdivisions or steps within each general category. Further, the institutions have set up salary advancement within and between grades to provide financial reward for increasing competence.[15] The aim of this policy is to provide greater recognition for those who pursue a career in nursing service, and, just as importantly, to improve the quality of care by retaining expert practitioners in their specialty.

To retain nurses in practice, reduce turnovers, and provide reasonable and needed incentives for nurses to continue in direct care activities, we recommend that:

> 3. *Health management administrators and clinical directors of nursing service build on current improvements in starting salaries to create a strong reward system for remaining in clinical practice by developing schedules of substantially increasing salary levels for experienced nurses functioning in advanced capacities.*

Because the profession must develop a long-term view of nursing practice, as well as underscore the need for increased professional competence, we feel that the present undifferentiated approach to clinical nursing skill should be revised. The personnel policies of all health care facilities should provide for advancement opportunities and commensurate financial remuneration. We recommend that:

> 4. *Personnel policies in all health care facilities should be so designed that they:*
> a. *Differentiate levels of responsibility in accord with the concepts of staff nurse, clinical nurse, and master clinician with appropriate intermediate grades. These levels should be designed according to the content of the position and the clinical proficiency required for competent performance;*
> b. *Provide for promotion granted on the basis of acquisition of the knowledge and demonstrated competence to perform in a given position.*

The last portion of the above recommendation stems from our findings during the on-site visits. We discovered that some health care facilities define promotional opportunities solely on the basis of time in grade or on formal educational achievements. While there are reasons for recognizing longevity and additional course work, the primary basis for advancement in nursing practice should be demonstrated knowledge and competence, whether attained through formal education, self-study, or experience.

For the effect of new salary and career advancement policies to be felt, however, there must be corrective action to alter the day-to-day problems related to nursing practice. In Chapter Four, we cited evidence that nurses spend perhaps 50 to 75 percent of their time in non-nursing activities, while patient care is frequently provided by unskilled personnel. In essence, we must take steps that will ensure that nurses have the opportunity to provide the highest quality of patient care. This entails a systematic examination and redirection of health care practices. Nurses must be released from non-nursing functions to concentrate on their unique professional contributions. Similarly, non-nursing personnel should take over every appropriate activity to ensure that the patient is given the best possible combination of services. We recommend that:

> 5. *Health management administrators and clinical directors of nursing service establish conditions to promote optimum opportunity for excellence in nursing practice by providing such elements as sufficient staff to develop and execute a personal care plan for each individual, the opportunity to discharge appropriate nursing functions in client teaching, counseling, and rehabilitation, and the surveillance and evaluation of the nursing plan for care.*

If we are to achieve full excellence in the humane delivery of health care, it will be through the proper discharge of functions by qualified personnel who have the time to function as they know they should. A constant state of crisis and shortage is debilitating to the profession—and intolerable from the standpoint of the client. In the long run, we must use nurses to their fullest professional capacity or our health care system will be in severe danger of failing.

There are a host of specific short-term activities that can aid in the retention and reactivation of nurses. The federal government has provided funds to establish refresher courses for returning nurses, but there is some indication that the graduates of these programs quickly become turnover statistics, probably for the reasons outlined in this section.[16] More promising may be the in-service and continuing education programs. In some cases, these educational opportunities include financial assistance, educational leaves, grants-in-aid to offset loss of salary, and loan forgiveness features. All these programs are designed to prepare the individual nurse for increased responsibility, and for greater clinical competence.

There is also evidence of growing flexibility in personnel policies. Married nurses, for example, have found that institutions are more willing to arrange schedules to coincide with family obligations. A number of health care facilities have adopted policies for maternity leaves, and still others have introduced, frequently with community cooperation, day care centers for preschool children of nurse mothers.[17]

Generally, our findings indicate that the retention and reactivation of nurses are largely influenced by the actions and policies of the local health facilities. Large-scale trends that affect the basic nurse supply, such as the number of women entering postsecondary institutions, the percentage choosing nursing as a field of study, and the attrition rate within programs, are problems that must be approached on national and state levels. At the same time, local initiatives that can sustain the community nurse supply are an essential corollary to national efforts. This commission recommends that:

> 6. *Local health care facilities adopt policies that provide for orientation and continuing education programs (including in-service and formal course work), more flexible employment policies respecting part-time work, maternity leaves, assistance for education to qualify for advancement, and leaves for education to encourage both the retention and reactivation of qualified practitioners.*

From this combination of economic and "fringe" benefits, we anticipate a realistic career enhancement program that will encourage capable nurses to remain in the work that first drew them into the field. The result should be improved patient care in all nursing areas.

RECRUITMENT OF NURSING STUDENTS

The conventional agencies for recruitment into all the professions are the academic institutions that prepare the future practitioners. In view of the magnitude of the current problems in nursing, the educational institutions need help in developing public understanding about the opportunities and needs for nursing students.

All the major health organizations, including the American Nurses' Association, the National League for Nursing, the American Medical Association, the American Hospital Association, and the American Public Health Association, have a crucial stake in recruiting future nursing students. At a time when greater numbers of entering students are needed simply to keep pace with population expansion, there is evidence that the proportion of high school graduates choosing nursing as a career is dropping—from 6 percent to 4.5 percent between 1956 and 1967.[18] Several explanations have been advanced for this decline. Some observers point to widening occupational choices for women; some suggest that the economic and other rewards in nursing are unattractive; and still others feel that information on nursing careers has not been well enough presented.

No matter how we attempt to interpret the immediate past, it is essential that prospective students have every opportunity to learn about the professional horizons within nursing, and the changing character of both the career and its rewards. We recommend that:

> 7. *The professional health organizations, including those in nursing, take responsibility individually and collectively for interpreting the characteristics of contemporary nursing to the public and direct their appropriate offices to undertake the task.*

While nursing has the primary responsibility of aiding educational institutions in recruitment efforts, other health professions should lend their aid and prestige to the promotion of careers in nursing. Many of the hospital associations have already become involved in these efforts. Ample opportunity remains for much greater collaboration in the effort to attract promising students into the profession.

Specific mention should be made of the crucial role played by high school guidance counselors in career selection. These individuals are often the major source of occupational information for secondary school students; the interaction of these counselors with students is a key factor in the survey of possible career choices. With the variety and ferment today in nursing education, there is little doubt that many of these counselors are unable to give complete and up-to-date information to young people. A number of state leagues and nursing associations have recognized this need and developed guides for counselors that provide current information on educational programs and career opportunities. As we anticipate the continued adjustment of programs based on recommendations by the state master planning committees, it will be incumbent on nursing to see that up-dated information is available to the counselor. We recommend that:

> 8. *State nurses' associations and state leagues for nursing undertake more effective dissemination of information to high school guidance counselors on the changing status of nursing, the opportunities for expanded clinical practice, the improving salary levels, and other career aspects of the profession.*

Even in the case of delayed career choice on the part of the student, better information at the secondary level can help provide a recognition of occupational alternatives, as well as basic knowledge about career attractiveness.

NEW SOURCES OF MANPOWER SUPPLY

Closely related to improved recruiting efforts is expansion of the manpower pool from which prospective nursing students are drawn. Research into student backgrounds indicates that the socioeconomic middle class supplies most of the personnel for the nursing profession.[19] This means that individuals at the extremes of the social scale—the disadvantaged and the highly advantaged—are underrepresented in nursing.[20]

In view of the growing need for more nurses, and the current decline in the choice of a nursing career among students who have traditionally supplied the bulk of the manpower, we must draw whole new groups into the recruitment effort.

One starting point is with the disadvantaged, many of whom are already acquainted with the health fields through employment as aides, attendants, and assistants. Today, more than half a million persons work in these capacities—a sizable resource even if only a small percentage could be recruited into nursing education programs each year.[21]

While there are merits in any plan to increase the opportunities for the disadvantaged, we must emphasize that their recruitment is not designed for social amelioration. Our goal is to provide quality input into nursing practice. The capabilities of many of these persons come to light only through job experience. Many administrators report that the disadvantaged, once productively employed, exhibit both the motivation and the intellectual capacity to assume far greater responsibility—responsibility that often requires additional education.[22] While some employers have capitalized on this discovery, many others have missed the opportunity to develop these talented individuals. With the recent move by labor organizations to adopt career ladders as a vital concept, there will be increasing pressure on health care facilities to look within their ranks to find likely candidates for professional training.[23]

Nursing has a fine record in fostering the recruitment of disadvantaged and minority groups into the profession. Now it has an unparalleled opportunity to seek ways in which nonprofessionals can qualify for advanced training. Frequently, talented subprofessionals who might otherwise qualify for advanced training will have deficiencies in such basic skills as English, mathematics, and science. It will require wide-scale cooperation on the part of many institutions to open paths by which these individuals can progress. In addition, many of these persons will need financial aid because they cannot forego their present income while pursuing formal education. Finally, we urge the profession to explore the possibilities for developing assistance plans that are proportional to achievement. The objective would be to reward individual excellence exhibited by these persons once they enter an educational program.

These proposals are not fanciful. A number of experimental projects are underway, including several in New York State, that provide remedial aid, financial assistance, and maintained earnings.[24] In view of this early experience, we recommend that:

> 9. *Public and private agencies and health facilities:*
> a. *Seek to identify talented individuals in lower job classifications who, despite probable shortcomings in formal education, display outstanding motivation, competence, and intelligence;*
> b. *Encourage and assist these individuals to obtain the necessary preparation to enter nursing education programs; and*
> c. *Provide scholarships and grants-in-aid to such individuals in amounts proportional to their demonstrated achievement.*

A second resource group for professional nursing consists of licensed practical or vocational nurses. Many times, these individuals are assigned to the supervision of patient units, a responsibility for which they are not formally trained. Indeed, this is a responsibility which they are not authorized to bear under most state laws.

There are nearly 300,000 practical nurses in the United States, with every indication that the number will increase as a result of state and federal support.[25] There is no doubt that many of the practicing vocational nurses exhibit broad technical competence, and many of them could qualify readily for registered nurse education programs.

Practical nurses should be encouraged to expand their knowledge and skill. In particular, they should be encouraged to complete educational programs leading to the registered nurse license. The Helene Fuld School of Nursing at the Hospital for Joint Diseases in New York City and Rancho Los Amigos in Downey, California, have developed specific programs to meet this need.[26] We encourage other institutions to explore similar policies, including flexible credit and instructional approaches. We recommend that:

> 10. *Institutions for nursing education develop career enhancement programs for licensed practical (vocational) nurses to furnish these individuals with added opportunities for professional growth through sequences leading to academic degrees and registered nurse licensure.*

Still another personnel resource for nursing can be found among the mature women who are preparing to enter the labor force for the first, or perhaps second, time. Actually, two distinct groups may be defined. The first consists of women who are graduates of liberal arts and science programs who may be attracted to the professional career in nursing; the second is composed of older women (who may or may not have had college experience) who have reared their families and are now exploring career possibilities.

In the first group, we find that there are more than 200,000 individuals who receive their baccalaureate degree each year in fields other than health. The approximately 10,000 graduates in the biological and physical sciences would seem a particularly promising group for recruitment. A total of 39,000 graduates in the social and psychological sciences represents another group that might identify strongly with the emerging profession of nursing. Some proportion of the liberal arts and science graduates might also be interested in the pursuit of a career sequence following their general college work.[27]

Today, only one institution, New York Medical College School of Nursing, offers a program tailored for these individuals, while other institutions provide some form of double baccalaureate preparation.[28] Nursing educators may find useful models in the Master of Arts in Teaching programs of the schools of education, or in other advanced programs in fields such as social work and library science, which provide first professional degrees at the graduate level. All these programs capitalize on the desire of the new college graduate to continue her education while she develops occupational expertise.[29]

Within the second group of women—the older and more mature persons— there is evidence of increasing motivation to reenter formal educational programs that prepare graduates for the professions.[30] Because American women marry at a younger age, and have their children earlier, there is a growing number of women, 35 and older, who can make a commitment of many years to an occupational choice. In the past, there have been problems in gaining institutional acceptance of readmission policies and specialized courses.[31] Our on-site visits indicated, however, that many of the emerging community college programs in nursing have been sought out by mature women. With effective communication and support policies, this group could constitute a significant resource for the nursing profession.[32]

To attract both the recent college graduate and the mature woman who might be interested in preparatory programs in nursing, we recommend that:

11. *Institutions for nursing education provide:*
a. *Expanded counseling services for mature individuals seeking initial entry into nursing preparatory programs; and*
b. *More preparatory programs for recent liberal arts and science graduates seeking a professional career in nursing.*

The final new source for nursing lies in the entry of men into the profession. While there are male nurses in the United States, men at present comprise less than 1 percent of the licensed registered nurses.[33] This situation seems particularly incongruous as one recalls periods in history when (as in the military orders of hospital knights) nursing was viewed as a male occupation.

Present developments in nursing, as well as general social trends away from sex-linked occupational definitions, may offer new opportunity for drawing a significant number of males into nursing. When nursing practice was essentially an intuitive art, it conformed to the social expectations of female behavior, i.e., giving tender, loving care. The growth of a scientific base to the profession alters these expectations. The emerging nursing role is suitable for anyone who can master it. Moreover, the recommended change in the economic picture should make it possible for heads of households, male or female, to support a family on a nurse's income.

From the public point of view, the recruitment of men into nursing could be highly important. There is no foreseeable event that can drastically change the patterns and extent of female participation in the work force. While the profession will probably experience greater retention and reactivation as the recommendations of this commission are implemented, women will still withdraw from employment because of childbirth and child-rearing. An enlarged body of men in the field could help to reduce these chronic problems of turnover and retention, and contribute to the long-term stability of the profession. There is also the possibility, if one looks at the field of professional education as an example, that men could hasten the economic and role changes that are needed to strengthen the nursing profession. The introduction of increased numbers of males into elementary and secondary teaching has materially aided in improving salaries and conditions for all educationists.

The broad-scale recruitment of men into nursing will, however, require innovative action by professional organizations as well as educational institutions. The effort is analogous to the current public efforts to increase the opportunities and employment of the disadvantaged. Action plans must be formed, specific recruitment goals set, and pressure maintained if there is to be any real increase in the number of male nurses. We recommend that:

> 12. Recruitment of men into nursing be fostered through efforts to modify the sex-linked occupational image of the profession by the national and state organizations, and the adoption of specific policies and goals to increase the percentage of males entering nursing preparatory programs by those institutions that offer them.

Through the intense effort to broaden the manpower pool for recruitment into nursing, not only the number of nurses, but also the socioeconomic composition of the profession, can be strengthened for the gain of both nursing and the general public.

LICENSURE AND CAREER PERFORMANCE

As nursing incorporates new and sophisticated therapies, the profession must provide adequate guarantees to the public that its practitioners function at a competent level. At present, all 50 states issue licenses for registered nurses. In eight states, however, the regulation is permissive and not mandatory. This has the effect of permitting any individual to perform the functions of a registered nurse so long as she does not attempt to represent herself as a licensed practitioner.

Such a situation may have been tolerable in the past when the functions of a nurse were relatively routine, required only a modest amount of judgment, and seldom involved danger for the patient. Today, with the changes in the levels of nursing responsibility, the absence of mandatory licensure represents a considerable potential hazard for the recipient of nursing care. Thus, it is for the protection of the patient that we recommend:

> 13. *All remaining states without mandatory licensure laws for registered nurses immediately adopt appropriate regulation to this effect.*

This commission recognizes that licensure laws have multiple effects. In addition to protecting the public from unqualified practitioners, there is the possibility that licensure can be used to limit the number of practitioners, or to seal off the license holder from public scrutiny. Most state boards of nursing have representation from outside the profession to ensure that licensure is not abused this way. It would be well, perhaps, to enlarge the representation of the general public on such boards. Traditionally, however, this has not been a problem in nursing, and there is little to suggest that it might become an issue.

The other kinds of problems involved in licensure, however, need more than passing examination. The fast-paced changes in health science raise the problem of assuring that nurses maintain their competence for practice. Laws governing health professions generally make no provision for a review of the licensed individual's capabilities. In nursing, this is now true in all states.

Of course, nurses are assessed by their clinical directors, but there is no legal provision for personal responsibility for continued growth in order to assure professional competency.

The conventional arrangement in those professions that provide for a periodic review of competence is proof of continuing study, both formal and informal. The introduction of such a concept into nursing practice, as currently proposed in the state of California, would require an individual to present evidence of such study as a requisite for relicensure.[34] We feel that some approach, perhaps similar to this, would provide an effective means for assuring professional competence. We recommend that:

> 14. *All state licensure laws for nursing be revised to require periodic review of the individual's qualifications for practice as a condition for license renewal.*

The current changes in the nursing role bear on another aspect of legislation affecting this field, particularly in relation to medicine. Flexibility in the nursing role and in professional performance is vital if optimum care is to be delivered. For this reason, licensure laws should not be designed to inhibit change.

Generally speaking, state laws and regulations attempt to define fundamental characteristics of practice in a field and do not attempt to assign particular procedures or interventions to one field or another. In the exceptional cases, however, where the language of laws and regulations is highly specific, the evolutionary process can encounter unnecessary difficulty. In such cases, the law can actually prevent the transfer of tasks from one professional group to another, and even the performance of procedures by individuals who are fully qualified by special training and experience.

The frequency of changes in role interpretation is evidenced by the number of joint professional statements on practice that have been promulgated in recent years. In 1968, for example, 18 states were represented by some 47 joint practice statements, and another 20 states had committees or advisory boards working on such statements. All of these involved nursing practice *vis-à-vis* other professions, the majority of them referring to nursing and medicine.[35]

These professional consultations contribute to the rational evolution of roles in the health care system while serving to safeguard the public's interest. As opportunities arise, however, the highly specific language of laws and regulations that impede constructive change should be altered. We recommend that:

> 15. *The language of licensing laws in nursing and medicine be couched in flexible terms to permit role evolution in accord with the emerging features of health service.*

A final consideration in licensure and professional performance is the recognition of differentiated levels of nursing practice. With the increasing gradations in nursing responsibility, particularly the emergence of the master clinician, we have heard suggestions that multiple levels of licensing should be invoked.

In some fields, such as professional education, there are multiple certifications. However, the health professions have held to the tradition of basic licensure followed by recognition of advanced levels through examination or review by professional bodies. The common example, of course, is the medical specialty board which certifies special competence beyond the M.D. degree.

Recently, nursing has initiated studies on the certification of individuals in advanced areas; this would seem to be a natural function for a designated arm of the professional organization.[36] The Academy of Nursing, still in the process of development, might well be the agency to assume such tasks as advanced certification. However, relationships must be worked out with the American Nurses' Association Division on Practice, which is currently examining certification. In any event, the procedures that are created should be reinforced by the personnel policies, accreditation standards, and other operating procedures so that there is uniform recognition for competence and advancement. We recommend that:

> 16. *In view of the emergence of advanced levels of clinical practice in nursing,*
> a. *A single license be retained for the registered nurse, and*
> b. *Advanced levels of nursing practice be recognized through:*

1. *Designation by approved bodies for such purposes, presumably the Academy of Nursing;*
2. *State licensing standards for health service units;*
3. *Qualifications for personnel specified in accreditation standards; and*
4. *Institutional personnel policies for appointments, promotion, and compensation.*

Proper application of certification procedures could supplement the needed changes in nursing roles and functions, and could aid in the speedy development of career perspectives. The interrelationship of these recommendations requires that nursing, through its professional organization, move to a quick resolution of the problems of advanced recognition.

PROFESSIONAL ORGANIZATION AND NURSING LEADERSHIP

In the past 20 years, nursing has emerged from a state of multiple, diffuse organization with scant resources to a more unified posture of strength. Part of this development was accomplished by a reduction process that combined several bodies into two national organizations: The American Nurses' Association and the National League for Nursing. The result has been a more unified voice for nursing and a clearer definition of the functions and responsibilities of the surviving organizations.

But nursing must continue the advance of recent years. It needs to study the structure and functions of the national organizations to project a consistent image to the public and to offer effective guidance to the thousands of American nurses. In recent months, the two national organizations have voluntarily begun to study their relationships and functions in an effort to increase the effectiveness of their work. We commend them for this willingness to examine themselves critically, and we recommend that:

17. *The national nursing organizations press forward in their current study of functions, structures, methods of representation, and interrelationships in order to determine:*
a. *Areas of overlap or duplication that could be eliminated;*
b. *Areas of need that are currently unmet; and*
c. *Areas or functions that could be transferred from one organization to another in light of changing systems and practices.*

The advances that nursing has made stem from the dedication of the leaders in the profession. They have been aided substantially, however, by the support of private foundations, public agencies, and ultimately the general public. Nursing has been quick to grasp the power of public support, and has capitalized on the relationship it enjoys by providing for representative lay leaders to serve on many policy-making and deliberative boards. In doing so, nursing anticipated many of the controversies that now abound concerning the responsiveness of all professions to the public good. Again, we commend nursing for this foresighted policy, and we recommend that:

> 18. *Nursing organizations, in effecting any of the changes that might come out of their current self-study, maintain their focus on responsiveness to health care consumers through the principle (perhaps unique to this profession) of providing for lay representation on their policy-making and deliberative boards.*

Not all is bright in the picture of the national nursing organizations, however. To realize the full potential of these groups, there must be far wider support among the individual members of the profession. According to current figures, approximately one-third of all registered nurses are members of the ANA. Because the NLN is directed toward community and institutional membership, an even smaller number of individual nurses belong. There is certainly room for several organizations to represent the varied interests and needs of American nurses, but in addition to membership in a group she feels is consonant with her particular interests, each nurse should be active in her primary professional organization.

It is a serious limitation to full professional recognition of nursing that so few of its practitioners belong to the national organizations. There must be serious in-depth study of this problem by the organizations—and serious self-study by nurses themselves. We recommend that:

> 19. *Individual nurses make a professional commitment to their organizations by joining and supporting one or more of them, at the same time ensuring that the organizations become more surely representative and more truly the designated spokesmen for nurses.*

In the final analysis, the development of the national nursing organizations is essential. It is true that the public can support education in nursing, help in career enhancement, and underwrite basic research. To the extent that the public gives this broad help, the profession can provide an increasingly large return in the form of improved health care.

Ultimately, however, it is nursing itself that is responsible for determining the bounds of its contribution to the public health. Each nurse assumes a personal, professional charge in entering the field. Accomplishment will be realized only through individual commitment and organizational excellence. The issue is still in doubt, in terms of true professional attainment. Only the nurses themselves hold the answer.

FOOTNOTES

1. See Chapter Three, pp. 50–53.

2. See Chapter Four, pp. 90–94.

3. Marshall, E. D. "Summary of SNA Annual Reports as of March 1969." New York: American Nurses' Association. November 7, 1969. pp. 51-57.

4. Interview, John Danielson, Evanston, Illinois, 6/5/69. American Nurses' Association. *ANA in Action.* 1:1:6. Spring, 1969. Interview, Hildegard Peplau, January 22, 1970.

5. "Projections of Registered Nurse Supply." Bethesda, Maryland: U. S. Public Health Service, Bureau of Health Professions Education and Manpower Training. 1969. Manuscript Draft. p. 27.

6. Marshall, E. D. and Moses, E. B. *RN's 1966: An Inventory of Registered Nurses.* New York: American Nurses' Association. 1969. p. 5.

7. *Technology and Manpower in the Health Service Industry 1965-75.* U. S. Department of Labor, Manpower Administration. May, 1967. p. 22.

8. Melbin, M. and Taub, D. L. "High Cost of Replacing Nurses." *Hospitals.* 40:20:112-122. October 16, 1966.

9. *Ibid.*

10. Argyris, C. *Personality and Organization: The Conflict Between System and the Individual.* New York: Harper & Brothers. 1957. See especially closing summary.

11. See Chapter Four, pp. 90–91.

12. American Nurses' Association. *Selected Provisions from State Nurses' Association Employment Standards as of January 1967.* New York: ANA Research and Statistics Department. pp. 6-30.

13. American Hospital Association. *Annual Reports—1969.* Chicago: American Hospital Association. 1969. p. 86.

14. Interview, Case Western Reserve University, 10/13/69; interview, Massachusetts General Hospital, 2/18/69; interview, Veterans Administration, Washington, D. C., 4/24/69.

15. *Ibid.*

16. Marshall, M. J. and Bruhn, J. G. "Refresher Courses and the Reactivation of Nurses." *Nursing Outlook.* 15:1:59-61. January, 1967. Mayberry, A. "Are Nurse Refresher Programs Worthwhile?" *Hospitals.* 41:11:95-100. June 1, 1967. Reese, D. E., and others. "How Many Caps Went On Again?" *Nursing Outlook.* 10:8:517-519. August, 1962.

17. The descriptions of personnel policies were derived from site interviews at Massachusetts General Hospital, 2/18/69; Case Western Reserve University, 10/13/69; and Beth Israel Hospital in New York, 4/29/69. A large number of articles appearing in hospital and nursing journals describe a wide variety of relevant policies. Examples of these are: Schechter, D. S. "Manpower for the Smaller Hospitals: Innovations in Training and Education." *Hospitals,* 41:11:55-58. June 1, 1967. Fanning, W. W. "Child-Care Nursing—One Hospital's Solution to the Nursing Shortage." *Hospital Topics.* 43: 12:51+. December, 1965. Davis, A. E. "Hospital-Provided Child Care Helps Nurse-Mothers Return to Work." *Hospital Topics.* 43:12:45+. December, 1965.

18. NCSNNE. Staff Study on Admissions and Graduations in Nursing Education Programs. Rochester, New York: 1969.

19. National League for Nursing Research and Development Department. "The Nurse Career Pattern Study: Biographical Data Reported by Entering Students, Fall, 1967." National League for Nursing Publication No. 19-1364. New York: The National League for Nursing. May, 1969. pp. 1-3.

20. *Ibid.* See also: Frackelton, D. L. and Faville, K. "Opportunities in Nursing for Disadvantaged Youth." *Nursing Outlook.* 14:4:26-28. April, 1966. Johnson, N. "Recruitment of Minority Groups—A Priority for National Student Nurses' Association." *Nursing Outlook.* 14:4:29-30. April, 1966.

21. American Nurses' Association. *Facts About Nursing, 1968 Edition.* New York: American Nurses' Association. 1968. p. 30.

22. Gotbaum, V. "Influence of the Labor Movement in Hospital Affairs." *Hospitals.* 44:1:73-74. January 1, 1970.

23. *Ibid.,* pp. 72–73.

24. Bumstead, R. "LPN Training: It's Worth the Struggle." *Training in Business and Industry.* 15:4:8-11. April, 1968. See also various publications of District Council 37, State, County and Municipal Employees, AFL-CIO, New York, New York, including "Intensive Training for the LPN Pin," "He'll Spread the Word About Our LPN Program," etc.

25. *Health Manpower 1966-75.* Washington, D. C.: U. S. Department of Labor, Bureau of Labor Statistics. Report No. 323. June, 1967. p. 24. American Nurses' Association. *Facts About Nursing, 1968 Edition., op. cit.,* pp. 164–167.

26. *Helene Fuld School of Nursing of the Hospital for Joint Diseases and Medical Center, 1968-1969.* New York: Helene Fuld School of Nursing. 1968. Feuer, H. D. "Operation Salvage." *Nursing Outlook.* 15:11:54. November, 1967. Mannion, S. E. "Upgrading LPN's to RN's." *Journal of Practical Nursing.* 19:9:31-32. September, 1969.

27. Simon, K. A. and Grant, W. V. *Digest of Educational Statistics, 1968 Edition.* Washington, D. C.: U. S. Government Printing Office. 1968. p. 87.

28. Site visit. New York Medical College. 11/25/68 and 5/1/69. For contrast, New York-Cornell Medical Center has a program for graduate nurses but the degree granted is BSN. Site visit 5/2/69.

29. According to the American Council on Education, for example, the number of women in graduate studies more than doubled between 1959 and 1967—from 97,373 to 236,000. The rate of increase exceeded the rate for men and is projected to reach 427,000 by 1975.

30. Riley, M. W. and Foner, A. *Aging and Society.* New York: Russell Sage Foundation. 1968. p. 44.

31. *American Women. Report of the President's Commission on the Status of Women. 1963.* Washington, D. C.: U. S. Government Printing Office. 1963. pp. 9-17. In spite of the publicity given to this report, relatively few institutions, such as the University of Minnesota, Northeastern University, and Radcliffe College, have established special programs for mature women.

32. *Ibid.*

33. American Nurses' Association. *Facts About Nursing, 1968 Edition., op. cit.,* p. 17.

34. Barham, Virginia, Nursing Education Consultant, State Board of Nurse Registration, California. Telephone interview, January 23, 1970.

35. "Summary Report of SNA Activities Related to Professional Aspects of Nursing Practice During 1968." New York: American Nurses' Association Research and Statistics Department. 1968. pp. 1 and 5.

36. *House of Delegates Reports, 1966-1968. 46th Annual Convention of the American Nurses' Association.* New York: American Nurses' Association. 1968. p. 58.

SEVEN
SUMMARY AND CONCLUSIONS

It is no easy task to draw together two and a half years' work in a few brief chapters of a final report. Even now, it is not easy to cut off portions of the investigation because there remain the nagging questions: Could we learn more? Might we uncover different information if we search longer? Of course, our answer must be couched in probabilities. If we have checked a sufficient number of sources, and if we have made allowance for varying points of view, then added investigation probably represents a diminished return on further investment of time and manpower. There is always the chance of the unexpected, but its likelihood is not very great.

In terms of setting a reasonable perspective for the study and its findings, however, we would like to share with the reader some of the concerns and reflections that abide with the staff and the commission concerning the protocols of the study. Then we will summarize our recommendations into a single conceptual framework and indicate the requirements and plans for implementation.

REFLECTIONS CONCERNING THIS STUDY

Perhaps the basic concern we might have about this study of a troubled profession lies in the choice of the commission to direct it and the staff to conduct the investigation. In general, an inquiry into a profession can be carried out in two ways. A study can be conducted by those who are expert because of their experience *within* the profession. Or, a project can be guided by investigators whose expertise comes from experience *outside* the particular profession.* For example, the researchers who wrote the *Survey of Dentistry*[1] or the Coggeshall report on *Planning for Medical Progress Through Education*[2] represent the within-profession model.

There are advantages in such an approach. The investigators know the field, they know many of the practitioners, and they are attuned to the nuances of differing points of view.

On the other hand, the Flexner report on *Medical Education in the United States and Canada*[3] and the Brown investigation of *Nursing for the Future*[4] are examples of the use of an outside investigator. There are plus factors in this approach as well. The researcher is not conditioned by the conventions and traditions of the profession, nor is he as influenced by the assigned status of various informants or the categorization of issues. In short, what is lost in efficiency by the need to "learn fresh" about the field may be made up in effectiveness by the objectivity of the observations. This commission chose the second approach — perhaps because of the old and deep controversies that are inherent in nursing. As one staff member put it, "We were too ignorant about nursing at the beginning for anyone to suggest that we were biased."

The independence and objectivity of the staff were complemented by the experience represented on the commission. Three of the 12 commissioners were nurses, with varying backgrounds and points of view. The remaining nine encompassed a diversity of professional interests including business, health administration, medicine, education, economics, sociology, and the public welfare. All had experience in serving on other investigative projects. Their active involvement in each phase of the study guaranteed a screening process to filter out any biases that were residual in our methods and techniques.

The study processes, through the deliberate involvement of many individuals and groups outside the nursing profession, ensured that the parochialism of an intragroup project would be avoided. Undoubtedly, this approach caused anxiety for those nurses who wondered why we should consult physicians, administrators, and lay people about nursing. We can reply only that we did consult these individuals *in addition to* nurse practitioners, nurse educators, and directors of nursing service. We felt that such an approach could widen the range of information and, at the same time, help to establish a consensus for later implementation of the commission's recommendations. By structuring the widest possible participation

* Ed. Note: For a general discussion of this difference in strategy, see Robert Merton, "Insiders and Outsiders: An Essay in the Sociology of Knowledge," a paper presented to the Centennial Convocation of Loyola University of Chicago, January, 1970.

at the outset, the staff attempted to minimize the likelihood of dissociation of any group that is essential for carrying out the needed changes in nursing. That is the reason for the involvement of non-nurses in the work of the commission, its staff, its advisors, and its discussants.

The long history of national nursing studies, dating back to 1923, is ample evidence that the profession alone cannot be expected to effect the recommendations enunciated for its improvement. Nursing must have the sympathy and help of the other health professions, the administrators of health facilities, and the general public. In a personal communication from Esther Lucile Brown, who directed the landmark 1948 study of nursing, the current staff was advised that the chief difference in thrust she saw between the two projects lay in her earlier assumption that nursing, together with an expanding economy, would be able to achieve the goals she outlined. Recognizing this had not been the case, she commended our effort to broaden the base for acceptance to ensure greater promise for action.

Limitations of the Study

While there are strengths and weaknesses in the fundamental decision to develop a study from within or without a profession, it is likewise true that any investigation has limitations that affect its validity and reliability. It would be improper not to point out the nature of these limitations so that later researchers, and the public, can recognize them.

One obvious limitation in our use of non-nurses in research is that they may fail to see or interpret essential variables in a complex situation. Recognizing this, the staff utilized several advisory panels during the course of the study. For example, the nursing panel aided us in delimiting problems, selecting sites for visitation, stating our findings, and eventually, in formulating our recommendations. To ensure a constant counterpoint, the health professions advisory panel was asked to examine the same kinds of questions, to react to all proposed findings and recommendations, and to interact with the staff and the nurse advisory panel on the later drafts of the recommendations.

The advisors were chosen by the staff in consultation with the commission, and in light of recommendations received from leaders of the several professions. However carefully one attempts to use such advisors, there are still limitations inherent in the system. The staff is obviously influenced by the consensus developed within and between groups; and we are bound by the experiences and capabilities of the individual and collective membership on the panels.

The nurse advisory panel, for example, included nurse educators and nursing service directors; its membership represented every current type of institution for preparatory nursing education. Moreover, the individual participants proved to be quite distinctive in their approach to, and resolution of, the problems that were identified. The health advisory panel encompassed administrators and physicians, as well as experienced investigators and scholars who had inquired into the nursing profession. In addition to these panels, which served throughout the study, there were invitational bodies and *ad hoc* groups that represented a wide range of backgrounds and expertise.

We attempted to make these advisory bodies broadly representative and individually excellent. We feel that the members have worked long and hard to make a contribution to the study, in an atmosphere free from slanting or adamant position-taking. Nevertheless, we must accept that one limitation to our study is the fact that we have used these small advisory groups and that they have had a strong and, we feel, positive influence on our investigation.

A second limitation exists in the selection of the sites for visitation. We queried our advisory panels and the commission, and searched the literature, for locations that the staff should study in person. Two criteria were advanced: examples of excellence in traditional practice or education; innovative essays in practice or education. Our initial list of suggestions numbered over 300 sites, a figure that was reduced to less than 150 through preliminary discussion with the advisory panels. After eliminating some duplication and finding that a number of projects were extensively reported already, we settled on approximately 100 sites to visit and study. Primarily, the limitation arose from our decisions to exclude some sites on the basis of available information. Thus, we may have missed the opportunity to see something important. In addition, in the cases of seeming redundancy, the choice was made on the basis of scheduling. That is, if two locations seemed to be involved in similar projects, then the staff was prone to choose the site nearer another institution for study so that the visits might be coordinated. With a small staff, a large number of locations, and limited time, this was a pragmatic approach, but one that surely affected somewhat the content of our report.

The third limitation lies in the type of material developed throughout the study—material that is useful for comparative, but not absolute, interpretation. Much of the information represents normative data that were lacking before. In the Nursing School Environments Inventory, for example, we were able to identify certain differences in the perceptions that students and faculties of various nursing schools had about their institutions. The greatest utility of this information will be found in years to come, however, when we discover whether the differences persist or whether changes within scores suggest changes within institutions. Likewise, much of the data on students, faculty, and institutions will have greater relevance at a later date when the commission's recommendations will have been invoked. Only then can we monitor effects to determine whether predicted results really have occurred.

In any event, one must be chary of attaching "good" and "bad" labels to normative data. If a certain percentage of nursing students extol the general excellence of their school, we must view this finding in light of what other nursing students think of their institutions; what other students, in other programs, say about their schools; and, perhaps, what other nursing students think of the same school after the passage of time.

Focus of the Study

One of the primary assumptions for this entire investigation is that there *are* problems in nursing. This is self-evident, but one unintended consequence of the search for what those problems are, and how to solve them, is that the emphasis of this study is related to what is wrong with nursing. Little attention has been focused on what is right in nursing. And there are many things that are right within this profession.

For example, nursing has cooperated with every development and new procedure in health care, oftentimes improvising methods and techniques to assist the physician and the administrator. This willingness of nurses to adapt is commendable. Too often, we overlook this quality when we consider the contributions of the health professions to patient care.

In common with all professions in the United States, nursing has generally lacked proportional representation from the minority groups within its body of students and practitioners. Earlier than most other groups, however, nursing sought this involvement, and the profession has made progress. As one example, in one three-year period, 1963 through 1965, the admission of Negroes to basic programs in nursing increased 30 percent.[5] Nursing is not, and cannot be, content with that achievement because the total number of black nurses is extremely small; but the change in direction is significant. Both the professional and student organizations have given prime urgency to the recruitment of the disadvantaged.

Another indication of the positive quality of American nursing is its very willingness to expose itself to outside study and analysis. Not every occupation or profession is so committed to renewal that it will welcome scrutiny that is bound to result in some criticism and suggestion for change. In this regard, nursing is unique among the American professions. Since 1923, a succession of studies, directed from both within and without the profession, has probed every aspect of practice and education. As one investigator put it, "Only college sophomores enrolled in general psychology courses have been studied more than the American nurses." Yet, the general cooperation of the schools and health facilities, and the individuals within them, was a striking feature throughout our exploration. There were times when an institution proved unwilling to take part in a survey, or perhaps to return a questionnaire, but this represented an insignificant problem.

One final comment must be made about the nursing profession. It is well enough to say that nurses cooperated willingly with our study staff. It is also important to point out that members of the profession never encroached beyond bounds in any attempt to sway the findings or recommendations of the study. Brown commented on this willingness to let facts speak for themselves when she mentioned, "Only once did members of the [nursing] profession attempt, through other than directly requested means, to influence the report."[6] Our experience in this regard was even more limited. Never did groups or organizations try to bring pressure on the report. Some individual nurses, of course, relished the opportunity to tell us what the report should say, but then at the very outset of our work one hospital administrator offered to write the entire report personally because he knew what the "facts" were going to be. Needless to say, we declined his kind proposal—as we declined the platforms of the few individual nurses who knew what the answers should be in advance of hearing the questions.

Atmosphere of the Study

Whatever other characteristics this study has exhibited, one hallmark has been our effort to avoid emotionalism. This does not mean that the commission and staff are unconcerned and aloof. It does mean that there are issues and problems that have become so charged with individual and organizational feeling that only psychological distance can permit real objectivity.

Some terms, like "professional" and "technical" nurses and "career ladders," have developed connotations that obscure the real world to which the terms refer. As Korzybski has pointed out, "The word is not the thing."[7] We have attempted to follow his dictate and concentrate on the real situation and not the label.

At the same time, we have sought to hear every point of view, even when it was presented emotionally. When observers charged that the commission and staff were alternately pro- and anti-nursing, we had some small assurance that we were treading a path between the extremes. We did not seek out the middle—only the avoidance of the edges. Some of our discussants, after the opportunity to say all the emotional things they had wanted to express for years, then displayed an admirable willingness to look at data dispassionately and even change their personal convictions. Perhaps these occasions alone were reason enough for the use of outside investigators in this inquiry.

A SUMMARY OF THE RESULTS

While the preceding chapters have presented the detailed set of recommendations, along with a discussion of findings, it may be useful to suggest one conceptual framework for all the specific proposals. We believe that the many recommendations for change in nursing can be seen in terms of four priorities:

    A. *Increased research into the practice of nursing and the education of nurses;*

    B. *Improved educational systems and curricula based on the results of that research;*

    C. *Clarification of roles and practice conjointly with other health professions to ensure the delivery of optimum care; and*

    D. *Increased financial support for nurses and for nursing to ensure adequate career opportunities that will attract and retain the number of individuals required for quality health care in the coming years.*

To suggest that changes in nursing begin with a dedication to the development of a greater knowledge base is hardly new. At the conclusion of her chapter on "The Future Role of the Professional Nurse," Brown cites the former Surgeon General in saying, "The nursing profession will make its best contribution only when it is organized to work with the public and to find its place in the team of allied professional groups. Its organization must be such as to promote research in nursing as a part of the overall health program. It must set up new channels through which new ideas can be received, evaluated, and used."[8]

This was true in 1948. It is still true today. There is a woeful lack of knowledge about the science of nursing practice and the outcomes of nursing intervention. In some areas, we have observed impressive gains. As mentioned in Chapter Four, practitioners do know more about such specialties as cardiac care nursing, and new roles for nurses in pediatric and ambulatory care. However, this is only the beginning of what we should know in order to ensure optimum nursing care for all patients. It is not sufficient that nurses act or refrain from acting on the basis of intuition or art. To practice without much more knowledge is to run the danger that Flexner emphasized in his assessment of medicine, ". . . such an expedient is to be regarded as a makeshift that asks of the sick a sacrifice that must not be required of them a moment longer than is necessary."[9]

There must be strong commitment to the systematic study of nursing practice in terms of objective criteria. This research will permit us to make scientific judgments about those things that nurses do that make a difference; and then to discover new things that nurses could do which would further enhance patient condition, recovery, and rehabilitation. As Brown emphasized so strongly, "By every means at its disposal the nursing profession, collectively and individually, must take a positive position concerning itself and the significance of its function. It must be as unquestioning in that position as are the medical and legal professions, which assume that their existence—on a progressively higher level of competence—is a social necessity and act accordingly."[10]

Brown charged nursing with the responsibility to assume the burden of research into its own practice for the sake of improving the quality of patient care.
Then she went on to say, "If society is interested in its own welfare, it too must
share in recognition of the vital importance of nursing."[11] It is in the full understanding of this responsibility to aid nursing in its public service that our commission formulated the first of its central recommendations that:

> 1. *The federal Division of Nursing, the National Center for Health Services Research
> and Development, other government agencies, and private foundations appropriate
> grant funds or research contracts to investigate the impact of nursing practice on the
> quality, effectiveness, and economy of health care.*

While we look to the expansion of knowledge about nursing to come from
this fundamental commitment to research, the commission also sees a need for
basic reorganization in the educational institutions for nursing. Since 1923, national, regional, and state studies have pointed out the problems inherent in a
system of both collegiate and noncollegiate institutions that prepare nurses for
their professional careers. The single-purpose hospital school of nursing has had a
long and vital history in providing the majority of nurses for practice. Without
gainsaying the contribution of these schools, it is a fact that institutions, like
individuals, grow and change. Likewise, institutional patterns must be constantly
reexamined to ensure that they are meeting their purposes, and doing so efficiently.

Over the past ten years, forces have been at work to change the traditional
patterns of nursing education. The number of hospital schools of nursing has been
sharply reduced; the number of collegiate programs, particularly in the community
and junior colleges, has grown rapidly. The shift reflects both the expectations of
society and the realities of the economy. By the former, we mean that more and
more students and their parents look forward to 14 years of general education as
the norm for today's young person. By the latter, we submit that four out of five
hospital schools of nursing are privately funded, while nine out of ten of the emerging junior college programs are publicly supported. These facts are not mentioned
to suggest a preference for public schools over private institutions. However, it
is essential to understand that most of the private support in the case of the hospital
school comes in the form of additional costs to the patients. In contrast, public
support for community or junior colleges is spread across the entire tax base of the
state. Moreover, contrary to the traditional view that hospital school education is
less costly, Altman's study of the economics of such schools has shown that it is
questionable whether an equivalent education can be offered less expensively in
the private hospital school.[12]

One might be willing to let the competing schools play out the game in a
crescendo of social and economic clashes were it not for the fact that the problems

are too critical to be left unresolved. While the professional controversy has raged over the best form of institution for preparing nurses, the high school graduates have given their own response to the situation: a slight but steadily declining interest in going into nursing at all. While the number of employed registered nurses has grown at a faster rate than the population during the last decade, it is a fact that in recent years a steadily smaller percentage of graduating high school seniors have chosen nursing as a career. In part, this development reflects the societal norm we mentioned earlier. Parents and graduates look forward to more years of general education, and tend to defer all vocational choices longer. On the other hand, Altman found that the desire for general academic courses, combined with a widening choice in the occupational outlook for the female high school graduate, tended to reduce the attractiveness of hospital-based preparatory programs.

As important as these trends are for the future of nursing education, little hard data were available at the beginning of this study on differences between the various preparatory programs. As reported in Chapter Five, our Nursing School Environments Inventory confirmed the impression that students perceive their institutions quite differently. At the same time, an analysis of student achievement on licensure examinations in New York State disclosed as much variation within any one kind of program as between any two programs. From this, one can conclude that all nursing education should be strengthened, but that no preparatory program is incapable of providing qualified graduates.

In the face of this mixed evidence about student achievement, and in view of new and major societal trends, we feel that nursing education should be structured to offer the most incentive and the most reward for the student. The one clear way to accomplish this is to center the educational system within the overall pattern of higher education, that is, within the collegiate institutions. In this context, nursing students have enlarged social, economic, and educational opportunities—and access to continued career development with a minimum of confusion or delay.

To say that nursing education should take place in collegiate institutions does not exclude a number of the current hospital schools from fulfilling every requisite as institutions of higher education. They have qualified and dedicated faculty, excellent facilities, ample resources, and motivated students. Through our contacts with the regional accrediting associations, we have learned that it is possible for some of these institutions to apply for, and receive, accreditation as degree-granting institutions in their own right. We commend this approach as one possibility for preserving their historic past and continuing their contribution to quality health care. Each regional accrediting association has provisions for recognition, and each hospital school interested in this course would have to initiate contact with the appropriate association.

Most hospital schools, it is true, would find the academic and financial requirements of regional accreditation beyond their resources. It is imperative, however, that they work in close cooperation with institutions of higher education to effect interinstitutional arrangements that will guarantee a continuation of the excellent clinical teaching facilities that now exist in the hospitals. No hospital school should close, and no collegiate program should open, until planning bodies have assured that an orderly transfer of functions and facilities has been developed. It is in the best interest of the whole country to ensure that this is carried out with speed and with positive direction.

For these reasons, the commission proposes as the second of its central recommendations that:

> 2. *Each state have, or create, a master planning committee that will take nursing education under its purview, such committees to include representatives of nursing, education, other health professions, and the public, to recommend specific guidelines, means for implementation, and deadlines to ensure that nursing education is positioned in the mainstream of American educational patterns.*

Along with the efforts to restructure the patterns in nursing education, it is imperative that the other health professions begin work in concert to spell out the congruent roles that they must develop if quality care is to be provided.

Nursing has a great number of tasks ahead in terms of studying the curriculum for students; articulating the best fit between elements and levels of the new institutional pattern; and attempting to find the most functional, effective, and economic approaches for the development of future nurses. These are projects that the profession can complete only after it has resolved the questions about the roles and functions to be required of a nurse practitioner. In other words, we must determine the objectives of education before we can begin to arrange an optimum set of learning experiences.

There are some things we can predict with certainty about the future role of the nurse. It will undoubtedly be more complex, more broad, and more varied than it is today—and it will most likely involve far greater degrees of independent judgment and action. This role development will stem from the growth of population and the critical shortage of physicians. The public and the other health professions will demand that nurses be utilized at their highest possible level of practice. As indicated in Chapter Four, there are voices in the American Medical Association already proposing that one solution to the serious health problems of the American people lies in the prospect of 50 to 75 thousand nurses practicing medicine under the supervision of physicians.

Today, serious students of role and role theory emphasize that congruent, or counterpart, roles must be worked out in some mutually contributory manner if there is to be real agreement and cooperation. This means, simply, that one cannot develop a role for a nurse apart from that of a doctor. Just as important, in this day of team health care, one cannot describe the full role of a physician apart from that of a nurse. The wisest individuals in both professions have long known and acted upon this simple fact.

Over the past several years, a series of joint conferences, statements on practice, and clinical meetings have emerged to begin formalizing what, in earlier years, were individual and rather informal agreements. This commission believes that the best approach for optimizing health care through role reorganization is that which can be accomplished directly by the professions involved. In other words, nursing and medicine can work out their mutual role relationships through joint discussion. If the resolution of the current problems of health care and its delivery does not follow, then there will certainly be a demand for solution by fiat—most likely at the level of the federal government.

It is our concern that mechanisms be established now to provide the ready means for the planning and development of roles. In forming this proposal the commission looks to the several states as units in which trials of role innovation can be conducted, and expanded or rejected as a result of these experiences. Likewise, the commission sees strength in the interaction that can take place between the state and national committees with a free flow of ideas and data in both directions.

As the third of its central recommendations, the commission proposes that:

> 3. *A National Joint Practice Commission,* with state counterpart committees, be established between medicine and nursing to discuss and make recommendations concerning the congruent roles of the physician and the nurse in providing quality health care, with particular attention to the rise of the nurse clinician; the introduction of the physician's assistant; the increased activity of other professions and skills in areas long assumed to be the concern solely of the physician and/or the nurse.

The final consideration in the conceptual structure is the necessity to pay for change and improvement. For a long time nursing has been viewed most favorably by the public; at the same time, this combination of respect and affection has not been translated into strong financial support. Economists might well develop the theme that nursing has subsidized our entire health structure through wages unreceived and benefits unobtained. Likewise, our support of nursing education and its institutions has been marked by parsimony. The early hospital schools quite bluntly offered training in return for service, and the length of the current diploma program reflects not only the justified concern to provide clinical experience, but the companion desire to extract compensatory service from the trainee.

Certainly, this commission is not opposed to the concept of social return on expenditures for student education. We believe, however, that educational requirements should be for purposes of education and that any form of required service should be designed to lengthen the probability of career practice. For this reason, we favor such approaches as forgiveness features in scholarships and loans that encourage—not student practice—but continuation in professional practice for longer periods of time.

In recent years, the level of federal support for nursing (which seems to act as a general barometer of all support) has expanded markedly. From 1960 to 1968, there was an increase in federal aid of almost seven-fold. We must look to these figures in perspective, however. The current expenditure of approximately $81,000,000 for nursing is approximately one-and-a-half times the support for practical nursing and one-tenth the support for medicine, while the number of nursing schools, students, and practitioners is far larger than either of the other two groups.

However, the commission did not attempt to develop its financial recommendations on such comparisons. Rather, we examined the experience of the Health Manpower Act, the analyses of the Surgeon General's Consultant Group, the Program Review Committee Report for the Nurse Training Act, and the National Advisory Council on Nurse Training as well as our own surveys on the needs of nursing institutions. From this, we deduced the figures presented in Chapter Five calling for a minimum level of $110 million in federal support and a desirable level of $125 million for fiscal 1971. We would also expect gradual, but continuing, increases from that point.

Current indications suggest that actual federal expenditures will approximate the minimum rather than the desirable level for reasons that include defense expenditures, economic trends, and other priorities. The absolute importance of the health care system, and the place of nursing in the critical position of dispensing that care, require us to urge either the increase of the federal support level to the desirable amount, or the increase of state and private support to compensate for the difference. Lest this be seen as an impossible amount, it might be helpful to visualize this expanded funding as a proportional increase of approximately $105 per capita for each current nursing student.

If the nursing manpower needs are, indeed, real, and if there is any commitment on the part of the public to the advancement of the profession, then the figures and the support levels recommended here are most modest—less than one-third of the amount we currently appropriate for the removal of surplus commodities. The commodity of nursing is not surplus, and we must begin to recognize it as a scarce and valuable resource.

The fourth and last of the central recommendations of the commission deals with the development of needed aid for nursing and its institutions. We recommend that:

4. *Federal, regional, state, and local governments adopt measures for the increased support of nursing research and education. Priority should be given to construction grants, institutional grants, advanced traineeships, and research grants and contracts. Further, we recommend that private funds and foundations support nursing research and educational innovations where such activities are not publicly aided. We believe that a useful guide for the beginnings of such a financial aid program would be in the amounts and distribution of funds authorized by Congress for fiscal 1970, with proportional increases from other public and private agencies.*

If this general concept of increased research, restructured patterns for education, planned role development, and general financial support for nursing and nursing education is adopted, then the century-old record of problems and inadequacies in nursing can be altered. Once there is acceptance of these central recommendations, the many proposals in each of the study areas will proceed logically and easily.

While these recommended changes will place a great burden for adjustment on nursing and the other health professions, they represent our best guarantee that nursing can begin to gird itself, along with the other components of the health care system, for the present demands that can only intensify in the years ahead. Nursing may well be the key to whether our entire system for health care will remain viable and responsive to the requirements it faces. It is essential, therefore, that the nation that makes those demands prove itself willing to support the efforts to meet them.

AN ABSTRACT FOR ACTION

Throughout this report, we have mentioned the numerous studies of nursing, independently conceived and independently conducted, that have resulted in generally similar recommendations. Likewise, we have pointed out that most of these recommendations have not been enacted; their contents have been noted, briefly discussed, frequently praised, and then filed away.

To allow this to happen once again would seem not only foolish, but, in light of our current health problems, catastrophic. Not to see that nursing works to its highest capacity, and not to ensure the greatest career potential for keeping nurses in practice, would affect not only this profession, but every other group that is marshaled in the cause of health. Inaction is not lack of action, but actually a further commitment to a retrograde movement that cannot be allowed to continue.

In 1948, Esther Lucile Brown incisively observed:

"Nurses have suffered frustration from the system of institutionalism within which they have worked and lived, and from insufficient sympathetic understanding by other health services and the public, as well as from their own inadequacies. This frustration has produced lack of self-confidence, which has transmitted itself to society. The public in turn has responded by continued disinterest or by sharp criticism. Thus a vicious circle has been instituted and perpetuated."[13]

Dr. Brown erred only in the sense that she felt that, by pointing out the nature of the problem, the nursing profession, buoyed by an expanding economy, could attain the objectives she presented. We know now, through the benefit of hindsight, that such a natural evolution is unlikely, and has not occurred. The forces of inertia are strong; the professional strength of nursing and its friends is too weak.

In such a situation, it is insufficient to detail the problems of nursing, to document a series of findings, to present a set of recommendations, and then to retire gracefully from the scene. It is necessary to propose a plan for implementation as well, a plan that can mobilize the forces for change in constructive ways.

The importance of concrete planning can be underscored when one considers the nature of the recommendations that have been presented. The greatest difficulties in nursing simply do not lend themselves to simplistic solutions. Otherwise, easy solutions would have been found long ago. In the present study, we have suggested the necessity for research into the basic practice of nursing. It will take time to develop answers to questions concerning the nature and effects of nursing practice, but support must start now. In the same way, the establishment of state master planning committees requires individual action by each state, with long-term benefits to be derived from the intercommunication of recommendations, action, and results. A final illustration lies in the need to set up the Joint Practice Commissions, which again requires time, patience, and great resolve. These things cannot happen quickly; they will not happen without dedicated and unremitting work on the part of some agency.

Of course, there are some things that can be accomplished immediately. Health care facilities can examine career compensation schedules and can bring more flexibility into employment and scheduling to attract inactive nurses back into practice. Even here, information and evaluation exchange would be helpful. And this kind of communication would be facilitated by the existence of an agency committed to the realization of this commission's recommendations.

In view of the short- and long-term implications of this study, the commission charged the staff with developing plans to ensure that these recommendations are enacted, or, from growing wisdom and experience, to spearhead alternative approaches to attain results more effectively. In response, the staff formulated an abstract for action that includes both immediate and continued phases.

The staff and commission held a series of regional meetings—13 conferences in seven locations—that served to announce these findings and recommendations.

The same meetings invited discussion, questions, and comments on those recommendations as well as suggestions for initial steps at implementation. To these meetings were invited leaders of the nursing profession, service, and education, and likewise decision-makers from the ranks of medicine, health management, government, third-party payers, other health professions and organizations, and the representatives of consumers, sometimes known in other contexts as patients.

These meetings provided the beginning of dialogue on a much enlarged base. They also represented the completion of the initial charge to both commission and staff for a short-term action plan. This approach does not, however, represent the termination of the implementation phase.

Proposals have been drafted and efforts are currently underway to acquire support for a continuing agency that would persevere for some years to accomplish the commission recommendations. This agency and its directing body would be designated as the successor to the commission and would strive for the ends that have been proposed here. The continuation of an independent and objective body, committed to the advancement of health care through the improvement of nursing practice, could be our one assurance that the year 2000 will not see just one more link in the long chain of nursing studies that are filled with "sound and fury—signifying nothing."

CONCLUSION

During the months of this study, the commission and staff have lived with the problems, the frustrations, and the triumphs of our American health system. In particular, we have become intimately acquainted with the history and the disappointments, as well as the great joys, of nursing. Out of this has come the recognition that nursing is not only important, but crucial to the future of health care in America.

Yet nursing has been and is a troubled occupation. It is an occupation that fails in every characteristic to achieve the status of a full profession, despite the fact that its best practitioners are professional in every sense of that word. It is an occupation that has never controlled its own destiny, but has suffered severe consequences when it has failed to meet the demands imposed by our society. It is an occupation fraught with paradox and promise—and it holds within itself the key to whether or not the vast majority of our people will receive quality health care.

Nursing cannot continue to be the stepchild of the health professions. In the concluding chapter of her report in 1948, Brown spoke prophetically when she said:

"Only when abiding conviction of social worth replaces lack of self-confidence, negativism, and carping comment, will that climate of opinion be created whereby nursing can move forward to greater selectivity of personnel and to a level of nursing care that bespeak growth and development for the nurse herself and more and better health service for society."[14]

Conditions have changed since she wrote those words—but not sufficiently. Meanwhile the nature and extent of our problems have deepened. This time, neither the public nor nursing can afford to fail. We must provide the means by which nursing can succeed. Furthermore, nursing must avail itself of fresh resources and use them. Nursing must take the opportunity afforded by these recommendations, capitalize on them, and emerge as a full profession, dedicated and capable. Any less achievement will represent less than optimum health care for all Americans, in all likelihood, for generations to come. Reveille sounds not for nursing alone, but for all those who want American society to enjoy the promise of the best health care, sensitively and humanely dispensed.

FOOTNOTES

1. Hollinshead, B. *The Survey of Dentistry*. Washington, D. C.: The American Council on Education. 1961.
2. Coggeshall, L. T. *Planning for Medical Progress Through Education*. Evanston, Illinois: The Association of American Medical Colleges. 1965.
3. Flexner, A. *Medical Education in the United States and Canada*. Boston: D. B. Updike, The Merrymount Press. 1960.
4. Brown, E. L. *Nursing for the Future*. New York: Russell Sage Foundation. 1948.
5. American Nurses' Association. *Facts About Nursing, 1967 Edition*. New York: American Nurses' Association. 1967. p. 91.
6. Brown, E. L., *op. cit.*, p. 14.
7. Korzybski, A. *Science and Sanity: An Introduction to Non-Aristotelian Systems and General Semantics*. Lancaster, Pa.: Science Press. 1933.
8. Brown, E. L., *op. cit.*, p. 100.
9. Flexner, A., *op. cit.*, p. 26.
10. Brown, E. L., *op. cit.*, p. 198.
11. *Ibid.*
12. Altman, S. H. "The Structure of Nursing Education and Its Impact on Supply." A preliminary draft of a report developed under U.S.P.H.S. Contract No. PH 108-67-204, "Economic Analysis of the Supply of Nurses." The preliminary draft was kindly supplied to our staff by Professor Altman for their use in data analysis. The final report will be publicly available.
13. Brown, E. L., *op. cit.*, p. 198.
14. *Ibid.*

GLOSSARY
OF TERMS

ACADEMY OF NURSING   That group of nurses charged with the formal recognition of advanced levels of clinical expertise among nurse practitioners as well as other functions assigned by the profession.

ADVANCED PLACEMENT   The practice of testing academic competence in a field, such as English or biology, and placing the student in advanced courses on the basis of indicated achievement of elementary course material.

AHA   American Hospital Association

AMA   American Medical Association

ANA   American Nurses' Association

ANF   American Nurses' Foundation

CHALLENGE EXAMINATION   An examination measuring knowledge in a field of study that can be the basis for granting exemption from, or credit for, an academic course without the requirement of additional formal class sessions.

CLINICAL NURSE   Middle levels or steps of nursing practice attained by demonstrating increasing competence in providing leadership for the nursing team and contributing significant clinical nursing skills to the patient care team.

CONTINUING EDUCATION   A formalized learning experience or sequence designed to enlarge the knowledge or skills of practitioners who have completed preparatory sequences. As distinct from in-service education, administration is normally in the hands of professional bodies or educational institutions rather than those of the employer.

DISTRIBUTIVE CARE   That area of concentration in nursing practice which emphasizes prevention of disease and maintenance of health and is largely directed toward continuous care of persons not confined to health care institutions.

DIVISION OF NURSING   A division of the U.S. Department of Health, Education, and Welfare that gives leadership in nursing practice and research, seeks to increase the number of nurses prepared for leadership positions, and provides a wide range of technical assistance designed to augment·and improve nursing services throughout the country.

EPISODIC CARE   That area of concentration in nursing practice which emphasizes the curative and restorative aspect of nursing and which usually involves patients with diagnosed disease, either acute or chronic.

ERIC   Educational Research Information Center. A national information system making available results from current educational research through a network of documentation centers.

HEALTH CORE CURRICULUM   A central body of basic knowledge, understanding, and skill that should be commonly known to all recognized health practitioners.

HEALTH MANPOWER ACT   Federal legislation enacted for the purpose of improving programs preparing nurses and other health professionals and allied health professional personnel through aid to students and support of preparatory institutions.

IN-SERVICE EDUCATION   A program administered by the employer that is designed to upgrade the knowledge or skills of the agency's own employees.

JOINT PRACTICE COMMISSION   That group of health professionals, nationally and in each state, charged with defining, through collaborative discussion and decision, the congruent roles of the providers of health care.

MANDATORY LICENSURE   A legal requirement that no individual may perform the functions of a professional nurse, or use that title, until he satisfies the appropriate state regulatory agency of his competence to practice and has been granted the agency's official sanction.

MASTER CLINICIAN   Advanced level of practice attained through clinical experience, additional study, and designation by an Academy of Nursing (or other group empowered to do so) which involves the demonstrated ability to make significant contributions to patient care through independent nursing judgments and scientifically based participation in the patient's therapeutic regimen.

NATIONAL CENTER FOR HEALTH SERVICES RESEARCH AND DEVELOPMENT   An agency that serves as the federal focus for health services research and development. The center supports, conducts, and fosters a national program of research, development, and demonstration projects addressed to major problems of health services, facilities, and technical equipment.

NURSE TRAINING ACT   Federal legislation enacted for the purpose of "increasing the supply of well-prepared nurses in the United States through a program of Federal assistance to schools of nursing and students of nursing."

NURSING SCHOOLS ENVIRONMENT INVENTORY   A survey instrument specially developed for this study (based on the Medical School Environment Inventory formulated by the Association of American Medical Schools) which records the perceptions of students and faculty to a variety of factors which exist in their individual educational environments.

STAFF NURSE   A beginning practice designation for graduates of all nursing preparatory programs that encompasses levels or steps attained by demonstration of increasing proficiency in the provision of nursing care.

STATE MASTER PLANNING COMMITTEE   That group, composed of representatives of the public, nursing, other health professions, and education, charged specifically with developing and establishing guidelines for implementing the commission's recommendations concerning institutions for nursing education.

UNIT MANAGER   An administrator at the ward or unit level who assists the nurse and/or the physician in providing an effective therapeutic regimen. A unit manager may be responsible to either hospital administration or nursing administration.

WARD CLERK   A clerical assistant to health care professionals (usually at the ward or unit level in health agencies).